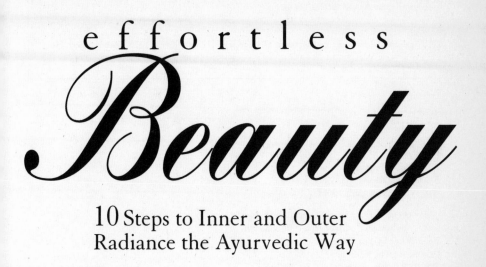

effortless Beauty

10 Steps to Inner and Outer Radiance the Ayurvedic Way

DR. HELEN M. THOMAS
AND NANCY PAULINE BRUNING

A Lynn Sonberg Book

PERIGEE

Most Perigee Books are available at special quantity discounts for bulk purchases for sales promotions, premiums, fund-raising, or educational use. Special books or book excerpts can also be created to fit specific needs.

For details, write to Special Markets, The Berkley Publishing Group, 375 Hudson Street, New York, New York 10014.

A Perigee Book
Published by The Berkley Publishing Group
A division of Penguin Putnam Inc.
375 Hudson Street
New York, New York 10014

Copyright © 1999 by Lynn Sonberg Book Associates
Cover photograph by Grace Huang Photography
Book design by Lisa Stokes
Cover design by Jill Boltin
Cover photo copyright © by Grace Huang
Illustrations/line drawings courtesy of the author

First edition: May 1999

Published simultaneously in Canada.

The Penguin Putnam Inc. World Wide Web site address is http://www.penguinputnam.com

Library of Congress Cataloging-in-Publication Data

Thomas, Helen M.
    Effortless beauty : 10 steps to inner and outer radiance the
Ayurvedic way / Helen M. Thomas and Nancy Pauline Bruning.
      p. cm.
    "A Lynn Sonberg book."
    ISBN 0-399-52501-7
    1. Beauty, Personal.   2. Medicine, Ayurvedic.   3. Health.
I. Bruning, Nancy. II. Title.
RA776.98.T46 1999
613—dc21
                                 98-50175
                                    CIP

Printed in the United States of America

10 9 8 7 6 5 4 3 2 1

This book is not intended to take the place of medical advice from a trained medical professional. Readers are advised to consult a physician or other qualified health professional before making any major changes in their diets or before acting on any of the information or advice in this book. If you have a medical condition, such as diabetes, please follow your physician or health-care professional's dietary and other guidelines and consult with him or her before acting on any of the information or advice in this book. The publisher assumes no responsibility for any health, welfare, or subsequent damage that might be incurred from the use of these materials.

I would like to dedicate this book to my aunt Liz Burke—her inner beauty speaks true testimony to the power of love; and especially to my husband, Craig Thomas, for recognizing my beauty every day.

—Helen Thomas

I would like to dedicate this book to my mother, Anne Marie, and to my yoga teacher Betty Roi—both of whom contributed to this book in subtle and real ways; and to J. B., whose presence in my life awakens my beauty.

—Nancy Pauline Bruning

CONTENTS

PREFACE

WHO HASN'T HEARD THE ADAGE "YOU HAVE TO SUFFER TO be beautiful"? Although looking good generally reflects an inner health in mind and body, and that takes some effort, it doesn't have to be a joyless grind.

Ayurveda, the original mind-body-spirit health system offers pleasurable, effective ways to be more beautiful on the inside as well as the outside. Every day you enjoy moments of spa-like luxury as you incorporate foods and practices that taste delicious and smell great as they make you feel wonderful and look great. You will learn how to turn your home into a relaxing, rejuvenating oasis for a day or a long weekend of beauty treatments that would cost hundreds of dollars a day at a professional spa. Ayurvedic practices and treatment are simple yet effective. You work with nature to achieve inner balance, vitality, and longevity—and in the process have better skin, healthier hair, more confidence and sex appeal, and a toned, supple body that tips the scales at your ideal weight.

The great photographer Francesco Scavullo recently said, "There are many types of beauty." He ought to know—for decades he has met and photographed the most beautiful, dynamic women of the world, including Liz Taylor, Brooke Shields, Verushka, Diana Vreeland, and Janis Joplin. Not all would be considered to be conventionally beautiful, but they all have found a way to express their true selves through the way they look.

While magazines and TV try to sell you an unachievable one-size-fits-all standard of beauty, the truth is that beauty comes in all shapes and sizes.

Ayurveda recognizes three different basic body types and shows you how you can live up to your individual potential through specific rejuvenating, purifying, and anti-aging techniques, practices, recipes, and products you make yourself from natural ingredients.

What makes our beauty and weight-control program so effortless is the secret of its success: you are working with the rhythm, flow, and unchanging principles of Nature, and with *your own* nature—not against it. With Ayurveda, you can reach your goals without artificial chemicals, without depriving yourself of delicious foods, and without forcing yourself to follow an exercise program that is unnatural for you and doesn't feel good.

Ayurveda, a Sanskrit word that means "knowledge of life and longevity," is based on principles and rhythms found in nature. It is not just a weight-loss plan or skin-care program. It is a way of life that makes use of daily and seasonal lifestyle practices (including diet, yoga, and meditation), healing herbs, purification therapies, and a life-affirming mental attitude.

At first glance, some Ayurvedic practices may seem exotic, foreign, or downright old-fashioned; however, they are actually universal, timeless, and as useful now as they were thousands of years ago. Fortunately, Ayurveda is flexible enough to accommodate today's lifestyles and needs. An experienced chiropractor, I began studying Ayurveda in 1987 because I was searching for a way to broaden and deepen my knowledge of human health and my ability to help people. Since then I have practiced Ayurveda myself and used it with thousands of patients since 1987. I know what works and what doesn't under a wide variety of circumstances.

I have found that even people who exercise regularly, eat a "well-balanced," low-fat diet, take vitamin supplements, and use expensive skin care products still don't look or feel their best. In spite of their efforts, something is still missing—they are not paying attention to their inner lives of mind and spirit. They are out of sync with their own rhythms and the universal rhythms of Nature. They lack connection and deep understanding of their inner selves and their outer world and an understanding of what true beauty is. Daily, monthly, and seasonal Ayurvedic practices nurture the whole person and provide tools to make those connections and reach that understanding.

As a health practitioner, I have always wanted to broaden and deepen my understanding of human health and expand my ability to reach and help people. That's why when Lynn Sonberg asked me to write a book about

Ayurvedic beauty I jumped at the chance. I had previously written a book with Nancy Pauline Bruning, called *Ayurveda: The A–Z Guide to Healing Techniques from Ancient India*. That was a marvelous experience for both of us, and we decided to team up again to produce this second book.

Once again, working as a team has been fun, educational, revealing—a marvelous journey for both of us. We discovered things about ourselves and about each other and learned how deep and meaningful and multidimensional a seemingly superficial topic as beauty can be.

I learned that Nancy, an established and distinguished author of seventeen books, most of them about natural or alternative therapies, worked briefly as a teen fashion model. A natural beauty and a brainy blonde, she eventually rebelled against the heavy makeup and the stringent dieting: although she weighed 124 pounds and was nearly 5'10" tall, her modeling agency wanted her to lose another fifteen pounds. She spent the next twenty-plus years relying on her youth and genetic good fortune, writing books that focused on what natural medicine could do to maintain and restore health. And she practiced what she preached, eating mostly whole natural foods, exercising regularly, practicing yoga, and meditating. But now that she has reached the age of fifty, thanks to this book, she realizes that doing the "natural thing" doesn't mean "doing nothing" about maintaining an attractive physical appearance and that natural medicine is also a safe, effective treatment for what ails you cosmetically. Having added Ayurveda to her repertoire, she says she's never felt better—and from head to toe, looks at least ten years younger than her age.

In working on this book and expanding my repertoire of health and beauty tools, I too have been transformed mentally and physically. Thanks to two babies and a hectic high-pressure professional life, I fell into the health professional's quagmire of caring for everyone else first. I never considered myself to be a beauty, so I have not paid that much attention to my appearance. I was unhappy about carrying a few extra pounds, but that was just part of who I thought I was. This book has forced me to reevaluate all of that.

Because I have been incorporating Ayurvedic practices and products into my life, I am reaping inner and outer rewards. I have noticed a huge improvement in my complexion. My skin feels much smoother since I have been using a cleanser based on chickpea powder. The lines on my face have become more shallow, thanks to the application of a moisturizer made of lime juice and honey. Nancy says my skin positively glows! I am more aware of what causes me to put on extra pounds and can control my weight better. Just as important, I am feeling the joy of nurturing myself. I am able to bounce back from day-to-day adversities much more readily. I have learned that if the world isn't nurturing you, at least you can nurture yourself.

Thanks to Ayurvedic beauty treatments, my patients have noticed this change in me—and in themselves as well. One woman, who was considering having cosmetic surgery to correct her drooping eyelids, has found Ayurveda to be a knife-free alternative. The solution was as simple as applying honey to her eyelids, allowing it to dry in place overnight and rinsing it off in the morning. This has tightened up the excess skin enough that she has decided against surgery, at least for now. Another patient with a history of severe acne rosacea has responded beautifully to a simple three times a day cleansing with a mixture of chickpea powder and turmeric. For the first time in many years she is not embarrassed to be seen in public, and her self-confidence and self-esteem have soared.

The transformation doesn't end there. When you go to the farmer's market to buy a fresh avocado to make a facial mask, you take in the sights and smells of all the other fresh fruits and vegetables that have been lovingly and locally grown, you meet the growers, and you are in the open air, which is also an aspect of pursuing your own inner beauty. The simple reality of mixing your own beauty products from fresh ingredients puts you in touch with the natural world and gives you a richer, more intimate knowledge of the ingredients. Cutting the avocado, preparing the other ingredients, and then putting them on your face, is an intensely personal activity in which you interact with the ingredients in an intimate way—and it is a hugely different experience from buying something in a plastic bottle. The simple act of applying a rich oil to your skin and running your hands over your own body during self-massage gives you a deeper knowledge and appreciation of yourself.

In this book Nancy and I have combined our experiences, thoughts, and abilities to present Ayurveda's beauty secrets in a clear, streamlined, useful form. We show you how to integrate Ayurveda into your everyday life and use it safely and effectively to nurture your inner self and cultivate outer beauty.

Ayurveda is a complete and holistic system that recognizes that each person is a unique individual, with a mind, body, and spirit that are intertwined. Outer beauty is a reflection of inner beauty, and a beauty regimen is not something you do for a half hour in your bathroom; it's something you practice twenty-four hours, every day, inwardly and outwardly. We all have the power to heal ourselves and let our beauty shine through for all to feel and see. It is our belief and hope that the information in this book will help you guide that power, enabling you to live a longer life, brimming with natural health, energy, happiness, and effortless beauty.

INTRODUCTION

Beauty from the Inside Out

WHAT IS BEAUTY? WHY DO PEOPLE CARE ABOUT IT? AND, JUST as importantly, how do you get it? These questions are at the heart of the Ayurvedic approach to beauty. The answers can have a profound effect on your life.

Beauty is difficult to define, because beauty standards vary from culture to culture and from era to era—and even from year to year. Poets and philosophers have struggled in vain to conquer this beguiling subject. From plucked eyebrows and ruby red lips to spiked hair and pierced navels, from rolls of fat and ample thighs to the anorexic waif look, from elongated necks and skulls to scarification and tattoos, from corseted waists and buxom bosoms to bound feet too deformed to walk on—women have been striving and continue to strive to measure up. Though astonishing in their diversity, beauty standards are inherently limiting. And they often involve a heroic amount of effort and discomfort.

Ayurveda does just the opposite—it expands the possibilities of beauty, helping you find and cultivate true beauty in yourself, in others, and in the world around you. In Ayurveda, beauty is neither a mask that you hide behind, nor someone else's idea, nor the latest trend. It is the outer reflection of the inner you, so it is ultimately honest, individual, and timeless.

As my patients have discovered, the Ayurvedic tools and techniques used to cultivate beauty are effortless in the sense that their actions are going with the flow of nature—not against it. The practices involve discipline, but it is discipline tempered with a great deal of pleasure. These practices are enjoyable themselves—eating good food, inhaling delicious aromas, enjoying oil massages—but there's more. Ayurveda's unique perspective helps you see yourself in a fresh, new light and provides you with the joy and fulfillment of making a commitment to yourself that exemplifies the love you feel for yourself and your body.

Why do we care about beauty? Why do so many of my patients come in with complaints not only about fatigue, digestive problems, and insomnia but also about pimples and wrinkles, too many bad hair days, and stubborn pounds that are ruining their enjoyment of life? Are they being obsessive or narcissistic? Not necessarily. We humans have sought physical beauty and delighted in its blessings since the dawn of our existence. The urge to be thought beautiful and desirable, to groom and decorate and embellish ourselves to achieve that goal, stems from a deep, primal need to be noticed, accepted, and loved.

Our parents, grandparents, foster parents, adopted parents, mentors, and dear friends are the first reflections of our beauty. The sublime gaze of a beloved mirrors to us the inner and outer beauty of our true self. The adoring look in their eyes when they watch us move through life is the seed of inspiration for our own inner journey. Once it has been planted, we water that seed each time we look at ourselves and see something we recognize as beauty. In our most important times in life we steal a glimpse of that beauty: Satisfied, self-assured, we walk down the aisle, accept the diploma, or make a presentation. Indeed, attractive people tend to be hired more often, be promoted, and have sweethearts. Are they self-assured because they know they are attractive, or are they attractive because they radiate confidence, happiness, and self-assurance? The answer to this chicken-or-egg question is: Both.

Ayurveda offers a liberating approach to beauty, one that serves the needs of women of different ages and different natural gifts. At the beginning of her career, Sophia Loren was told that her mouth was too large, her nose too long, her chin and lips too broad—but that still the sum of her parts were "somehow beautiful." She never fit the current standard of beauty, and now that she is a woman "of a certain age," she has achieved yet another kind of beauty that is very different from her youthful appeal. In her book *Women and Beauty*, Loren points out that whereas the beauty of youth is unconscious, mature beauty is knowing and sophisticated, richer and more complex. In her book, she shares with us her greatest beauty secret: her unfailing self-confidence. "If you can use your mind as well as you use a powder puff," she writes, "you will become more truly beautiful." Her message and that of Ayurveda is: **You can attain beauty because beauty is already inside you.**

THE AYURVEDIC WAY TO HEALTH AND BEAUTY

Ayurveda believes that it is natural to be vibrant and beautiful—and it is natural to *want* to be that way. Ayurveda recognizes that the desire to be attractive is deeply ingrained in the human psyche and that connecting to your own beauty is to face the primordial mystery: Who am I? Your beauty is a crucial aspect of your feelings of self-worth, an expression of who you really are. Through its unique process of body typing, Ayurveda introduces you to yourself, shows you your potential, and then helps you make the most of what nature gave you.

Ayurveda is a six-thousand-year-old healing and disease prevention system from India. It is gaining in popularity, in part through the immense talent and success of one of my teachers, Deepak Chopra. What few people realize is that Ayurveda is also a *beauty system*. Unlike Western conventional medicine and cosmetics, it does not distinguish the pursuit of inner and outer health from the pursuit of inner and outer beauty. It is also unique in its emphasis on natural methods of body care and rejuvenation.

Does health create beauty or beauty create health? Another chicken-and-egg question. Again, the answer is: Both. Just as mind and body are so inextricably connected as to be one and the same thing, so are health and beauty intrinsically related. People who are healthy and vital in body, mind, and spirit are also beautiful in body, mind, and spirit. Poor skin, premature wrinkles, dull hair, bad breath or body odor, low energy, depression, extreme overweight or underweight are the outer signs of illness within. But glowing, radiant skin, shiny hair, sparkling eyes, vitality, cheerfulness, and ideal weight are outward signs of inner health. Whatever supports health also supports true beauty. In achieving one, you achieve both.

In addition, when you actively pursue the true beauty that resides within, you experience deep knowing and satisfaction that radiates from within. Connecting with this feeling nourishes you so deeply that health becomes the effortless by-product. Radiant with energy, your skin, hair, and eyes gleam with the cream of your life juices, called *ojas* (OH-jas) in Sanskrit. No makeup, cream, or mask can substitute for this, your first step in discovering your inner beauty.

If beauty comes from within, why bother with creams, potions, and cosmetics at all? Because external beauty may be just the icing on the cake, but icing tastes wonderfully sweet! Artifice—makeup, hair color—and decoration—jewelry, fragrance—can certainly have a place in your total beauty picture. But they are just that: an illusion, an embellishment, an artful form of play. Experimenting with a new moisturizer, facial mask, or aromatic bath oil is fun. Even here, you can choose ingredients and materials that are in sync with nature, and in the process, achieve a more beautiful effect. Unlike commercial products, home-prepared Ayurveda products are not based on hype and unrealistic promises—"hope in a jar." They are devoid of fancy packaging that hikes up the price and generates unnecessary waste. Ayurveda uses natural ingredients that you can easily understand—many from your kitchen cabinet—that have been safely used for hundreds and thousands of years. The idea is not to go back to that time, but to reacquaint yourself with the wisdom of ancient traditions and bring them up to date—a blending of old and new, putting the best of both at your disposal. Just because you meditate to achieve inner peace doesn't mean you can't use mascara to enhance your outer beauty.

HOW TO USE THIS BOOK

We have arranged this book in a progressive, step-by-step program. We hope you will read it all the way through as you begin to acquaint yourself with the general principles of Ayurveda and how you can put them to use. Some of our recommendations will be a radical departure from your current life practices and even your worldview. Neither your mind nor your body likes to be shocked, so let the information sink in and then begin incorporating changes in your life gently and slowly. Evaluate your life and your needs, and use that as a guide in deciding how much you want to change. Someone who works a night job will need more rebalancing than someone who works a regular day job. Someone with a high-stress profession, a second career as a parent, or both will need more nurturing than someone with a more laid-back work life.

In the first chapter, "Step 1: What's Your Mind-Body Type?" you will learn about the basic concepts of Ayurveda, the Ayurvedic view of health and beauty, and the three *doshas* (DOH-shahs) that are the overall guide in tailoring Ayurvedic practices to the individual. Part of this first step is to take a self-test to determine your essential nature so that you can learn how to support well-being and beauty Ayurvedically and uncover any basic imbalances you are experiencing at this time.

Good digestion and a healthy metabolism are necessary for optimum health, inner radiance, and outer beauty, and the next chapter shows you how to take "Step 2: Nourishing Your Body." This is where you learn one of the most fundamental practices of Ayurveda—how to feed your body with food, herbs, and spices appropriate to your body type. In "Step 3: Nourishing Your Mind and Spirit," you will study ancient Ayurvedic techniques that feed your inner self. You'll learn how to calm and enliven your mind and spirit with deep relaxation, meditation, and yoga, and methods for pleasuring all five of your senses. "Step 4: A Beautiful Face Every Day" provides you with basic skin care techniques to maintain healthy skin and remedy problem skin. In "Step 5: Beauty Secrets for Skin and Hair" you learn how to take care of your body—skin, hair, hands, feet—and how to treat specific problems. In addition to basic skin and hair care these two chapters present a vast array of cosmetic products that you can make yourself from fresh natural ingredients—cleansers, moisturizers, scrubbers, massage oils. Together, Steps 2, 3, 4, and 5 provide you with a repertoire of effortless techniques and practices designed to rejuvenate your skin and other organs, prevent premature aging, prolong life, and foster spiritual and mental health for an inner glow.

The next three steps involve putting these practices to use in customized routines. Begin with "Step 6: Daily Spa Programs for Radiant Beauty"— basic plans for living every day the Ayurvedic way, in tune with the daily rhythms of nature. "Step 7: Once-a-Month Spa Program" shows you how to turn a long weekend into a mini-spa-like vacation to rejuvenate yourself inside and out. "Step 8: Seasonal Purification Program" is a more intensive purification and beautification spa experience designed to help you make a smooth transition between the seasons.

In "Step 9: Effortless Weight Control Program," we provide the best weight control program you'll ever find. You'll learn to establish realistic, reachable goals based on your specific body type, how to reduce cravings, boost metabolism, and achieve your ideal weight without dieting or counting calories. We also tell you the secret to using yoga to tone and firm thighs, hips, waist, and arms.

"Step 10: Cultivate Your Sexual Charisma" acknowledges that there's more to attractiveness than physical beauty and further helps you cultivate desirable inner qualities such as confidence, self-love, and self-respect that turn other people on. There's also a special section on how to improve your sex life.

Finally, in the last section of the book we have gathered together resources for herbs and other Ayurvedic remedies and practices mentioned in earlier sections. You'll also find books and other informational resources we recommend if you wish to deepen your knowledge and practice of Ayurveda. As you follow the Ayurvedic practices suggested in the daily, monthly, and yearly routines we provide in this book, you will be filling your life with effortless pleasures. Imagine greeting every day with a soothing massage, eating fresh, seasonal, deliciously spiced foods, and regularly taking time out to close your eyes, relax, and get in touch with your deepest self. As you will see, Ayurveda is a system of pleasures, not deprivations. It is your key to not only *looking* beautiful, but to *being* a beautiful person.

THE BEAUTY OF SANSKRIT

The beauty techniques in this book are based on Ayurvedic texts that were written in Sanskrit, the language of ancient India. This extinct language is now used only for sacred or scholarly writings. Although many of the original Sanskrit terms have survived the translation into English and are used by practitioners in talking and writing about Ayurveda, in our first book about Ayurveda, we kept the use of Sanskrit words to a minimum. We wanted to make Ayurveda accessible to as many people as possible and felt that using too many foreign words would be confusing in an introductory book written for a general audience.

However, in that book—and in this one—it is impossible to avoid Sanskrit words completely because sometimes there is simply no adequate translation into English, or the translation is awkward. One example is *dosha*, which means literally "that which has a fault" and is often translated as "governing principle." Other examples are the names of the three types of doshas, *vata* (VAH-tah), *pitta* (PIT-ah), and *kapha* (KAH-fah)—these have no translation at all. Another is *prakruti* (prah-KROO-tee), which some writers and practitioners translate as "constitution," or "body type," or "personality," or "biotype," or even "physio-psychological constitution." Some of these English equivalents are a mouthful without being quite accurate. Therefore, for practical reasons, in many instances we give a thorough explanation of the concept when it is first introduced and then use the much more precise Sanskrit term thereafter.

There is another reason to provide you with the Sanskrit term: Sanskrit is a beautiful, poetic, musical language. Which yoga position makes you feel more beautiful: *Standing Forward Bend* or *Uttanasana*? So in keeping with the spirit of this book, we supply many more Sanskrit words along with the English equivalent than in our earlier work. You will soon feel comfortable referring to the doshas and your prakruti. And you will feel more lovely performing Uttanasana.

STEP 1

What's Your Mind-Body Type?

*T*HE FOUNDATION OF THE AYURVEDIC APPROACH TO HEALTH and beauty rests on determining your individual nature and body type—*prakruti* in Sanskrit. In my practice, I am inevitably asked the question "What am I?" In this chapter, you'll find a test that helps you answer that question for yourself, from an Ayurvedic point of view. Once you have determined your prakruti, we will help you determine whether you have any imbalances that are at the root of any beauty or health problems you may be having. We then explain how to choose the regimens and programs that are right for you in addressing your particular beauty concerns.

But first you need to have a basic understanding of the underlying philosophy of Ayurveda—how the five elements and three governing forces interact to create the fluctuating state of being that encompasses you, your world, and all of existence. Understanding how Ayurveda works enables you to see and cultivate beauty everywhere—including in yourself.

THE FUNDAMENTALS OF AYURVEDA

Ayurveda may seem strange or exotic at first, with its Sanskrit words used to describe a different way of looking at beauty and at the world in which beauty can unfold. But the basic concepts are really simple and easy to grasp: there are *five elements* from which everything is made and *three forces* that govern everything; when these three forces within us are balanced, we are free to be beautiful and healthy.

The Five Elements and the Three Doshas

Ayurveda recognizes five basic elements, or constituents, to be the smallest components to which anything can be reduced. They are air, space, fire, water, and earth. Everything in nature is composed of these five glorious, mysterious, essential components—including you.

Air is the Ayurvedic term for the gaseous form of matter.

Space (sometimes called "ether") is the expanse or area in which air is contained and through which it moves.

Fire is the radiant form of matter and is needed for any process of transformation, or "digestion."

Water is used to describe the liquid form of matter.

Earth is the solid form of matter and is responsible for groundedness and solidity.

The five elements, in infinite combinations and proportions, are the basis for all life-forms and things. They also constitute three forces, or *doshas* in Sanskrit, that govern all the functions of the body, mind, and universe. The three doshas, or governing principles, are called *vata, pitta,* and *kapha.* Each dosha has its own set of characteristics, which arise out of the elements from which they are made. This includes the physical and emotional characteristics and personality traits of people, as well as of everything else. For example, there are vata, pitta, and kapha kinds of flowers, people, houses, music, foods, trees, birds, and bees, as well as times of day and seasons. There are vata, pitta, and kapha skin, hair, nails, weight tendencies, and so on.

You will learn more about the doshas and the characteristics they bring to individuals later in this chapter. Following are brief introductory descriptions of the doshas:

Vata is composed of the elements air and space; air, the dominant element, is contained within the spaces and channels of the body. The vata in you governs any movement of your mind and body and the flow, circulation, and activities of the nervous system.

Pitta is composed of fire and water; fire, the main element, is contained within the protective waters of the body (such as digestive enzymes). Your pitta force governs your metabolism—the body processes involving heat, digestion, and hormones and biochemical reactions such as those required to produce energy.

Kapha is composed of earth and water; water, the main element, is contained within the body's mass, or earth. The kapha dosha in you governs your body's structure and tissues and maintains stability, cohesion, fluid balance, and biological strength.

Every person (and thing) contains all three doshas in varying proportions. However, usually one or two doshas predominate. Your individual constitution—the unique proportion of the three doshas that you were born with—is called your prakruti. Your prakruti is your true, essential nature. No dosha is inherently better than any other, and no proportion of doshas is more desirable than any other. You need them all and you need them to be in balance, as determined by your prakruti, in order to function and sustain health.

Within each person, the doshas are continually interacting with one another and with the doshas in all of nature. This interplay among the fundamental forces and components explains why people can have much in common but also have an endless variety of individual differences in the way they look, behave, and respond to their environment. The doshas in us help explain why you may be experiencing prematurely dry skin and wrinkles, why your friend has sensitive skin that breaks out in rashes from certain cosmetics or stress, and why your sister battles constantly to lose weight. These are innate tendencies for which creams and weight-loss diets offer only a superficial, temporary fix. However, by understanding your doshas, Ayurveda helps you treat the underlying imbalance that is the root cause of your complaints.

The idea that there are certain body types and personality types has also appeared in Western thinking. For example, in the area of weight control and body shape, people have been categorized as ectomorphs (lean and sinewy), mesomorphs (muscular), and endomorphs (soft and rounded). These categories roughly correspond to the vata, pitta, and kapha types, respectively. And the notion that individuals have differing innate vulnerabilities to certain diseases has also gained a foothold in modern medicine. Recently, a bestselling book was published that prescribed diets based on an individual's blood type. However, the concept of the doshas and their relation to health and beauty is much more holistic, integrated, subtle, and complex than any of the above ideas.

The doshas are abstract concepts, invisible themselves but evident everywhere you look once you are aware of them. Physicists can't fully explain the phenomena known as *gravity* and *magnetism*; yet we can see and feel their power to pull and push things around. So it is with the vata, pitta, and kapha forces.

Maintaining Balance and Beauty

Your doshas fluctuate by interacting with other doshas in the world— stress, food, pollution, tastes, colors, sounds, aromas, and changes in the seasons affect the doshas in different ways. For example, very hot and pungent spices aggravate pitta; but cold, light foods such as salads calm it down. As a result, health and beauty are locked together in a dynamic process of continual small compensatory adjustments.

This ability to affect the doshas is the underlying basis for Ayurvedic practices and therapies. You can experience this dynamism when you do balancing yoga poses, in which you can feel your physical body undergo subtle changes to maintain equilibrium. It is evident during meditation, in which your mind continually returns its attention to your mantra as thoughts and feelings draw it away. And it is at work after drinking an herbal tea that reduces your need to *absolutely* have that entire chocolate bar *right now*.

Your prakruti is your inherent, ideal condition. But because of the various influences on the doshas, your actual condition may not match this ideal. In Sanskrit there is a name for your current condition: *vikruti* (veh-KROO-tee). Although vikruti reflects your ability to adjust to life's influences and is always changing, it is best if these fluctuations remain minor ones. If the current proportion of your doshas differs significantly from your constitutional proportion, it indicates imbalances that in turn can lead to illness and a less attractive appearance. As you will see in the next chapter, good "digestion" is the key to maintaining and restoring your ideal proportion of the doshas—your prakruti.

The simple, entertaining, and enlightening self-test that follows allows you to decide which prakruti most closely expresses the essential you. Once you understand your prakruti, you have taken the first step toward a beauty and weight control program that is effortless because it is based on the love, understanding and high-quality care that you are giving to yourself. By determining your prakruti, you will discover the particular characteristics, tendencies, and potentials you are capable of fulfilling. Understanding who you are, why you are the way you are, and how outside influences affect you physically and emotionally familiarizes you with the positive and negative characteristics of your doshas. Rather than putting you in a box, such understanding is wonderfully liberating. Instead of judging yourself and others, wanting to change yourself or someone else to fit an impossible mold, you can develop a love and acceptance as well as a whole set of tools that allows you to encourage the most positive, beautiful aspects of your doshas to emerge.

SELF-TEST: DETERMINE YOUR MIND-BODY TYPE
(PRAKRUTI)

Your prakruti is a guideline to your natural state and your potential. This test will answer the question: What's your essential nature?

To take the test, on a blank piece of paper, make three columns with the letters V, P, and K at the top, one for each dosha. Then ask yourself each question, and respond with 0, 1, 2, or 3, in each column based on the following scale:

0 = Never or almost never, no
1 = Rarely, mild
2 = Sometimes, moderate
3 = Frequently, severe, yes

When finished, add up each column; the dosha with the highest number is the predominant dosha in your prakruti.

	VATA	PITTA	KAPHA
My skin is . . .	Dry, flaky, thin, rough, cool to touch	Oily, smooth, with freckles or moles, warm to touch, glowing	Oily, thick, smooth, soft to touch
*My complexion is . . .	Bluish	Red, ruddy, or yellowish	Pale
*My hair is . . .	Dry, brittle, thin, or coarse, brown, black	Fine and straight, blond, red, graying early or balding	Oily, thick, luxuriant, wavy, curly, dark
My eyes are . . .	Small, nervous, dry, black or brown	Sharp, bright, sensitive to light, gray or green, with a penetrating gaze	Big, calm, blue, with a loving gaze
My teeth are . . .	Big, crooked or protruding, healthy with thin, receding gums	Medium-sized, yellowish and soft, with tender gums	Strong and white with healthy gums
My lips are . . .	Dry, thin, dark red, or yellowish	Soft, pink, and firm, pale	Oily and smooth, large, thick
My bone structure is . . .	Slim, slight, prominent	Medium	Thick, solid, heavy
My height is . . .	Above or below average	Average	Average or tall
My muscles are . . .	Wiry, undeveloped	Moderately developed	Solid, stocky, well-developed
My weight is . . .	Below average, I lose weight easily	Medium, able to lose or gain weight	Above average, I gain weight easily

*When looking at these categories, take into consideration that in every ethnic group there is a natural range of shades and textures; some attributes may not apply to you.

	VATA	PITTA	KAPHA
Most of my fat is located . . .	Around my waist	Evenly over my body	Around the hips and thighs
My veins are . . .	Prominent	Somewhat visible	Not visible
My shoulders are . . .	Narrow and slope downward	Medium-sized	Broad, firm, developed
My hips are . . .	Narrow	Medium width	Wide
My hands are . . .	Small, dry, cool, with small, long fingers	Medium-sized, moist, warm, pink	Large, oily, cool, firm
My nails are . . .	Dry, rough, brittle, and break easily	Flexible, pink, and lustrous	Thick, smooth, shiny, and hard
My perspiration is . . .	Scanty with no odor	Heavy with strong odor	Moderate or heavy with pleasant odor
My lifestyle is . . .	Highly active	Active	Rather inactive
My appetite is . . .	Irregular, with skipped meals	Strong, must eat regular meals	Constant, but can skip meals
My sleep pattern is . . .	Irregular, light, interrupted, 5–7 hours a night	Sound and even, 6–8 hours a night	Prolonged and deep, difficult to wake up
My gait is . . .	Quick, short steps	Medium pace, purposeful	Slow and graceful
My energy or endurance is . . .	Low, energy comes in spurts, then need to rest	Well-managed	Good, long-lasting
My speech pattern is . . .	Fast, talkative	Precise, convincing	Slow, monotone, melodic

	VATA	PITTA	KAPHA
The pace of my activity is . . .	Fast	Medium speed, intense	Slow, steady
My sex drive is . . .	Either in very high or very low gear	Moderate frequency, but passionate and domineering	Infrequent, constant or cyclic, loyal and devoted
I dislike weather that is . . .	Cold, windy, dry	Hot, with strong sun	Cool and damp
I am . . .	Flexible, optimistic, lively, intuitive, enthusiastic, changeable, an initiator	Ambitious, practical, intense, motivated, perceptive, warm, friendly, independent, courageous, discriminating, a good leader, goal-oriented, competitive	Calm, peaceful, solicitous, resilient, content, loyal, slow, deliberate, relaxed, compassionate, patient, nurturing, stable
My memory is . . .	Quick to remember—and to forget	Average, clear, distinct	Slow to remember—and to forget
My thinking style is . . .	Restless, quick	Organized, efficient, accurate	Slow, methodical, exacting
I process information . . .	Quickly	At medium speed	Slowly
My creativity level is . . .	Filled with ideas, but tend to follow through poorly	Inventive in many areas, with good follow-through	Best in the field of business

	VATA	PITTA	KAPHA
Under stress I become . . .	Anxious, insecure, tense, and sigh and hyperventilate	Aggressive, angry, irritable, headachy, nauseated	Lethargic, dull, in denial
I dream of . . .	Activity, running, flying, frightening things	Violence, fire, anger, passion, the sun	Romance, sentimentality, water, and snow
When making decisions I am . . .	Unsure	Quick and decisive	Deliberate
Emotionally, I . . .	Worry, am anxious, moody, and emotional	Get angry and irritated easily	Stay calm, complacent, get angry slowly
I love . . .	Traveling, art, esoteric subjects	Sports, politics, luxury	Good food

Determining Your Dominant Dosha: Are You Vata, Pitta, or Kapha?

Once you have taken the test and added up each column, you can easily see which dosha is dominant: the one that has the highest score. As we said earlier, everyone is a combination of all three doshas, but in most people, one dosha: vata, pitta, or kapha takes center stage. It's quite possible that your scores will be close or equal for two of the doshas. This suggests a two-dosha type, meaning that you express qualities of your two leading doshas nearly equally. However, one dosha usually predominates, even though the difference may be small—thus, the fine distinction between pitta-vata and vata-pitta, between vata-kapha and kapha-vata, and between pitta-kapha and kapha-pitta. On the other hand, if the scores for all the doshas are nearly equal, you are a rarity—a three-dosha type. However, even in a three-dosha type one dosha usually edges out the others.

Because most people are combinations of all three doshas, at times you will exhibit characteristics of each. This can be confusing if you are a newcomer to Ayurveda. To help you get a better picture of the characteristics of the three doshas, read the following descriptions and see which fits you best:

Vata · If you have a vata-dominant prakruti, you are light, changeable, and unpredictable as the wind. You have a slight, thin build; a restless mind and body, and are a light sleeper. You move and think quickly, love excitement and change, go to sleep at different times every night, skip meals, and keep irregular habits in general. When in balance, you are cheerful, enthusiastic, resilient, charming, vibrant, vivacious, sensitive, full of imaginative ideas and creative energy, exhilarated and exhilarating to be around.

Pitta · If pitta predominates in your nature, you are intense and fiery, with a strong drive, self-control, and unforgettable, piercing eyes that are part of your mesmerizing personality. Of medium build and strength, you feel sharp hunger and thirst and get irritable and feel faint if you don't eat on time. Hot weather is not your friend. You tend to communicate through your skin—you blush and flush easily and are glowing and radiant when healthy and happy. When in balance, you are joyful, extremely creative, and have an enterprising character that enjoys challenges; you have a sharp intellect and you let everyone know it with your precise, articulate speech and rapier wit. You live by the clock and can't bear waiting or being delayed. You are a born leader and often take command of a situation (or feel that you should).

Kapha · This is the slow, grounded, solid, placid dosha. If you are a kapha type, you are earthy and heavy, with a full-bodied, gently curving figure and great endurance. People can get lost in your large, wide, thick-lashed eyes and are attracted to your welcoming, sensuous, serene demeanor. You generally act and think methodically because you need a long time to digest information. You digest food slowly, too. When in balance, you are calm, graceful, loving, nurturing, sympathetic, forgiving, and slow to anger. However, you seek comfort from eating and tend to be overweight. Have you ever joked that you gain weight just by looking at a chocolate sundae? If your prakruti is high in this dosha, you are slow to get out of bed in the morning, most strongly feel the need for a strong morning espresso, and tend to be generally sluggish.

WHERE ARE YOUR IMBALANCES?

Your prakruti, your essential nature, is an ideal state, and it is always in a state of flux because the doshas are influenced by everything in our inner and outer lives. One dosha—or two—can at any time become aggravated or excessive. As a result, its qualities become exaggerated, and the remaining doshas become overwhelmed and can't do their job. This in turn leads to a variety of symptoms that are characteristic of the exaggerated dosha— problem skin, weight problems, and poor health in general.

Often, your predominant dosha is the one that goes out of balance most easily. Thus your health and beauty complaints offer another clue to your basic nature. Check over the following lists and note which symptoms you tend to experience most often, or are experiencing now.

Your vata is aggravated if you . . .
- Have excessively dry, rough, flaky skin and chapped lips
- Dark circles or puffiness under your eyes
- Dandruff
- Suffer from insomnia or wake up at night
- Experience constipation, intestinal bloating, or gas
- Have low energy and poor stamina
- Are very sensitive to cold
- Bite your nails
- Have arthritis or stiff and painful joints
- Your eyes feel dry
- You have low appetite and have experienced recent weight loss or are underweight
- Feel tired, yet wired
- Are worried, anxious, fearful, or nervous
- Can't relax and are antsy or hyperactive or restless
- Have trouble concentrating
- Space out

Your pitta is aggravated if you . . .
- Have inflamed, irritated skin rashes or hives
- Have whiteheads
- Have stomach problems such as acid stomach, heartburn, or ulcer
- Wake up frequently and can't go back to sleep, have disturbing dreams, or night sweats
- Have bad breath
- Are very sensitive to heat and get hot flashes
- Get bloodshot eyes easily
- Have a sour body odor
- Feel weakness due to low blood sugar
- Experience food allergies
- Get angry, irritable, hostile
- Feel impatient and get frustrated easily
- Are critical of yourself and others
- Argue with others
- Are aggressive, bossy, and controlling

Your kapha is aggravated if you . . .
- Have excessively oily skin with blackheads or pimples
- Gain weight easily or are overweight
- Retain water and feel bloated
- Have sluggish digestion and food seems to "just sit in your stomach"
- Have low energy, sleep too much, feel very tired in the morning
- Remain drowsy or groggy during the day
- Experience mucus and congestion in your chest, throat, nose or sinuses
- Your thinking and reaction time are sluggish or dull
- Feel sadness or are depressed
- Procrastinate

Understanding Imbalances

Ayurveda is exquisitely logical. Notice that these symptoms of imbalance reflect the elements that comprise the affected dosha. For example, vata imbalances reflect the drying, airy, disruptive powers of the wind. Pitta imbalances reflect the burning action of fire. Kapha imbalances reflect the heaviness and stagnation of water.

What causes these imbalances to occur? Again, Ayurveda is quite logical in that it is based on the principle that "like increases like." Here's how this works: Activities, foods, and thoughts that have the same qualities as a particular dosha will "feed" or stimulate that dosha, and too many of them will overstimulate it. Therefore, if your prakruti is predominantly vata, you will experience imbalances from time to time when you work too hard, drink too much coffee, sleep irregularly, or are out and about in cold, dry weather.

The key to good health and good looks lies in maintaining and restoring the balance that is your genetic heritage. By balance, we don't mean trying to give yourself equal amounts of all three. Not only is that impossible— that would be going against your inborn nature—but it would be quite dull to have everyone so similar! The idea is to find the balance that is right for you, first by correcting any severe imbalances that exist now and then to maintain your new balanced condition by following the daily routine that's tailored to your prakruti. A more accurate term might be *stabilize* because we want to calm down the elevated dosha and rev up the quiescent ones.

Staying Balanced and Restoring Balance

Once you have determined the predominant dosha of your prakruti, you are ready to follow the rest of the program. You'll be able to follow our guidelines for nourishing your body (Step 2) as well as nourishing your mind and spirit (Step 3). Furthermore, you can determine the particular skin and hair care regimens and formulas suited to you individually (Steps 4 and 5). And you can decide which spa programs you will be following on a daily, monthly, and seasonal basis (Steps 4, 5, and 6). These programs help you maintain good health and vibrant good looks and prevent any problems to which your dosha might be prone. Your dosha also serves as a guide in following the weight control program (Step 9) and in cultivating your sexual charisma (Step 10).

Note that the doshas shade one another, and oftentimes a strong vata imbalance will create confusion. That's because vata leads the other doshas and thus can cause pitta-like or kapha-like symptoms when the underlying cause is really a vata imbalance. If your pitta or kapha appears to be out of balance but following a pitta- or kapha-based program doesn't help within a month, try the vata-balancing programs. Or consult a professional, experienced Ayurvedic practitioner for diagnosis and advice.

STEP 2

Nourishing Your Body

"*Y*OU ARE WHAT YOU EAT" HAS BECOME A CLICHÉ. BY now it's common knowledge that food provides the fuel and raw materials your body needs to maintain and repair itself. Still, this basic truth is one reason that after you determine your body type, the next step is to learn how to keep it well nourished so that you can more easily maintain or enhance your appearance. In this chapter we explain the principles behind the graceful and sensible Ayurvedic way of eating. After the comprehensive lists of the specific foods and cooking herbs appropriate to your dosha, you'll also find a guide to eating beautifully so the food you eat can be transformed into a more beautiful you. Next, we provide a section on the use of herbs and spices and finally a selection of recipes for basic Ayurvedic dishes and digestion-strengthening remedies.

In Ayurveda, however, it's not only *what* you eat that counts. It also matters *how* food is grown, prepared, served, eaten, digested, and assimilated. If the food you eat isn't itself healthy and delicious and in possession of its own kind of health and beauty, if you eat on the run or while under stress, then what you eat, no matter how nutritious, can't contribute much to your well-being, inner peace, and attractiveness, either.

Another unique aspect of the Ayurvedic view is that food—which includes herbs and spices—is classified according to its taste and other qualities, which correspond to the qualities of the three doshas. Vitamins, minerals, protein, fat, carbohydrate, fiber, calories all count, but there is so much more to food than those elements. Because Ayurveda considers other aspects of foods, eating and drinking appropriately for your body type is the foundation for achieving greater health, beauty, and control of your weight and shape.

Included in this chapter are lists of foods to emphasize and those to avoid. Even so, you'll find that this approach isn't limiting. You will not feel deprived of certain foods because Ayurveda helps you break free of the rut of eating the same foods day in and day out and relying on just a small selection of herbs and spices for seasoning. Ayurveda opens up a whole new world of delicious things to eat and drink that are beneficial, not detrimental, to your health and appearance.

THE IMPORTANCE OF GOOD DIGESTION

According to Ayurveda, digestion is the cornerstone of health and beauty because good digestion nourishes the body. Eating properly will make a big difference in your appearance and well-being—but these foods must also be properly digested and assimilated so that they can be distributed to all the cells of the body. The creators of Ayurveda observed that digestion is not just a matter of digestive enzymes breaking down food into its smallest physical molecules, but rather a complex interplay between mind and body.

Agni (AHG-nee): Your digestive fire. One of the most fundamental concepts in Ayurveda is that of *agni*. Agni is the digestive and metabolic "fire" produced by the doshas that grabs the essence of nourishment from food (and, as you'll see later, from your feelings and thoughts and the experiences of all your five senses) and transforms it into a form that your body can use. Through the heat of agni, various tissues of the body produce secretions, metabolic reactions, and other processes needed to create energy, maintain and repair the body tissues including the skin, and enable your immune system to destroy harmful organisms and toxins. Agni is needed to form *ojas*.

Ojas (OH-jas): The substance that maintains life. *Ojas* is the by-product of a healthy, efficient, contented physiology. It is the "juice" that remains after food has been properly digested and assimilated. When you are producing ojas, it means all your organs have an integrated vitality, and you are receiving the nourishment your mind and body need. Your whole being hums with good vibrations because you are producing and feeling bliss, not emotional or physical discomfort or dissatisfaction. Ojas is the creamy, healthy look you see in your reflection when you are really taking care of yourself. However, when your agni isn't working properly, you don't produce ojas. That's when what you take in turns into *ama* and trouble starts.

Ama (AH-mah): Accumulated toxins. *Ama* arises from improperly digested toxic particles that clog the channels in your body through which food, blood, lymph, oxygen, nutrients, and energy travel. Ama toxicity accumulates wherever there is a weakness in the body, and this will allow a genetic predisposition to overtake you, and create or maintain disease. While Ayurveda offers ways you can cleanse the body of ama, it's best to prevent it from forming in the first place. A sure sign of an ama problem is blemished skin, a coated tongue, or weight problems.

Malas (MAH-lahs): Waste products. *Malas* are the waste products of your body and include urine, feces, mucus, and sweat. Eliminating waste is crucial to good health, but dosha imbalances stifle the flow of the malas, creating a toxic internal environment. If you are not eliminating malas, it means you are accumulating ama somewhere in your system.

Prana (PRAH-nah): The life-force. Another key concept in Ayurveda is *prana*, the life-force that enters the body at birth and travels through all the parts of the body until it leaves at the moment of death.

FOOD AND YOUR DOSHAS

〇～

Foods not only contain material sustenance such as protein, fat, carbohydrate, and vitamins. They also contain packets of intelligence, or information, some of which are analyzed by our ability to taste. Therefore, in Ayurveda, the primary way that you choose the right foods for you is by their taste.

In addition to the six tastes, foods are characterized according to six other qualities—heavy, light, oily, dry/drying, hot/heating, cold/cooling—which also affect the doshas and must be taken into consideration. Generally, doshas are unbalanced by foods that have the same qualities as the dosha and are balanced by those which have the opposite qualities. Here's how the six tastes—sweet, sour, salty, bitter, pungent, astringent—and the six qualities affect the doshas:

HOW THE SIX TASTES AND SIX QUALITIES AFFECT THE DOSHA

VATA	PITTA	KAPHA
Balanced by Sweet★, sour, salty Heavy, oily, hot	*Balanced by* Sweet★, bitter, astringent Heavy, oily, cold	*Balanced by* Pungent, bitter, astringent Light, dry, hot
Unbalanced by Bitter, astringent, pungent Light, dry, cold	*Unbalanced by* Sour, pungent, salty Light, dry, hot	*Unbalanced by* Sweet★, salty, sour Heavy, oily, cold

Common Examples

　　　Sweet: Sugar★, milk, cream, butter, rice, honey, bread, pasta

　　　Sour: Yogurt, lemon, plums, and other sour fruits, vinegar, cheese

　　　Salty: Salt, seaweed, foods that have salt added

　Pungent: Spicy foods and spices such as chilis, cayenne and black pepper, ginger, cumin

　　　Bitter: Spinach and other bitter green leafy vegetables, endive, chicory

Astringent: Beans, lentils, pomegranates, apples, pears, cabbage, rhubarb

Heavy: Cheese, yogurt, wheat products, brown rice, red meat, sesame oil

Light: Barley, corn, spinach, apples, mung beans, basmati rice, chicken, sunflower oil

Oily: Dairy products, fatty foods, oils, most nuts, eggs

Dry/drying: Barley, corn, potatoes, beans, millet, pears

Hot/heating: Heated food and drinks, sesame oil, meat, onions, eggs

Cold/cooling: Refrigerated or iced food and drink, milk, sunflower oil, coconut, wheat

(*Note: Refined, white sugar is to be avoided by all doshas; Sucanat, a new product made from the juice of organic sugarcane, is acceptable as a sugar substitute. If you have diabetes, you should consult your doctor before including Sucanat in your diet.)

FOOD GUIDELINES

What the above chart tells us is that there are certain tastes and characteristics that make specific foods more appropriate for one dosha than for others. The following lists provide you with a handy guide to use in choosing your everyday foods according to your predominant dosha. Following these guidelines helps you stay in balance and makes it easier to care for your skin, hair, and body and to control your weight.

When choosing foods from the lists, aim for foods that are in season and grown in your local area. If you are two-doshic (you have approximately equal amounts of two doshas), you can choose from both food groups when you are in balance. For example, a pitta–vata can eat from both the pitta and vata food lists. However, no food is completely forbidden. If you are a vata, you can sometimes eat popcorn, just as pittas can have garlic, and kaphas can have a double-fudge brownie on special occasions. You can enjoy any food from all of these lists *occasionally*.

Remember to give yourself time to adjust to these new tastes in your life. Often when things don't appeal to your taste buds, it's because you've become habituated to a limited palate. Introducing all six tastes, in proportions appropriate for your dosha, restores your true metabolic alignment and your delight in your sense of taste.

Vata Foods

Use these guidelines for eating if:
- your prakruti is predominantly vata, or
- you have symptoms of an aggravated vata, such as dry skin and hair, insomnia, or low energy.

General principles:

Eat and drink primarily foods that stabilize vata: warm foods and beverages, oily foods, foods that taste predominantly sweet, sour, or salty. Avoid foods that aggravate vata: light, dry foods, cold foods and drinks, and foods that taste predominantly pungent (spicy hot), bitter, or astringent. Eat regular meals, and avoid skipping meals or fasting.

Vegetables:

Avoid raw vegetables. Emphasize sweet potatoes, parsley, cilantro, beets, carrots, seaweed, avocados. Eat in moderation: peas, green beans, artichokes, squash, turnips, okra, watercress, cauliflower, cucumbers, asparagus, celery, chard, spinach. Eat small amounts of the following: brussels sprouts, broccoli, cabbage, zucchini, onions. You may eat mung beans, tofu, kidney beans, lima beans, and chickpeas in moderation, but avoid pinto beans, lentils, split peas, and soybeans.

Fruits:

Emphasize lemons, limes, grapefruit, grapes, prunes, strawberries, raspberries, cherries, pineapples, dates, figs, mangoes, papayas. In moderation, you may eat pears, bananas, oranges, peaches, apples (cooked), pomegranates, apricots, plums, and persimmons. Avoid cranberries, melons, and other dried fruits.

Grains:

Emphasize rice, wheat, and oats. Eat moderate amounts of barley, corn, millet, buckwheat, rye, and quinoa (especially avoid these in popped or puffed form).

Nuts, seeds, and oils:

All nuts and oils are acceptable, but eat sunflower seeds, coconuts, and pumpkin seeds in moderation.

Animal foods (nonvegetarians):
All dairy products (except ice cream), eggs, fish, and shellfish can be eaten. Eat cheese, chicken, turkey, lamb, and beef in moderation; avoid pork.

Sweeteners:
Date sugar and fructose, barley malt, rice syrup, raw unrefined sugar; use Sucanat, fruit sugar, and honey (orange blossom only) in moderation; avoid white sugar.

Pitta Foods

Use these guidelines for eating if:
- your prakruti is predominantly pitta, or
- you have symptoms of an aggravated pitta, such as irritated skin, bad breath, offensive perspiration, or a bad temper.

General principles:
Eat and drink primarily foods that stabilize pitta: cool foods and drinks and foods that taste predominantly sweet, bitter, and astringent. Reduce foods that increase your natural heat, such as foods that are predominantly pungent (spicy), sour, or salty.

Vegetables:
Emphasize asparagus, pumpkin, cucumber, broccoli, cauliflower, avocado, celery, lettuce, zucchini, okra, green beans, mushrooms, alfalfa sprouts, cilantro, sunflower sprouts, brussels sprouts, cabbage, peas, aduki beans, mung beans, lima beans, and tofu. Eat in moderation bell peppers, parsley, squash, corn, carrots, cooked onions, chard, spinach, beets, sweet potatoes, turnips, radishes, seaweed, watercress, split peas, soybeans, kidney beans, chickpeas, lentils.

Fruits:
Emphasize apples, cranberries, prunes, grapes, cherries, melons, coconut, pineapples, plums, pears, pomegranates. Eat in moderation raspberries, oranges, plums, mangoes, bananas, lemons, limes, papayas, persimmons. Avoid grapefruit.

Grains:
Emphasize wheat, oats, barley, white rice, and quinoa. Eat moderate amounts of millet, brown rice, corn, rye, buckwheat.

Nuts, seeds, and oils:
Emphasize sunflower seeds, coconut, ghee★★, butter, coconut oil; use in moderation pumpkin seeds, pine nuts, sesame seeds, peanuts, and olive, soy, sunflower, safflower, corn oils. Avoid cashews, walnuts, almonds, pecans, filberts, and sesame, almond, and peanut oil.

Animal foods (nonvegetarians):
Emphasize milk, cottage cheese, and cheese; use in moderation chicken, turkey, egg white, fish. Avoid sour cream, yogurt, buttermilk, ice cream, lamb, shellfish, pork, beef, and eggs.

Sweeteners:
Maple syrup, fructose, rice syrup, barley malt, raw unrefined sugar; use Sucanat, molasses and honey (wildflower only) in moderation; avoid white sugar.

Kapha Foods

Use these guidelines for eating if:
- your prakruti is predominantly kapha, or
- you have symptoms of an aggravated kapha, such as oily skin and acne, overweight, excessive sleeping

General principles:
Your diet should consist primarily of foods and beverages that stabilize kapha and are stimulating: choose foods that are light, dry, and warm, and that taste primarily pungent (spicy), bitter, or astringent. Avoid overeating in general and specifically foods and beverages that aggravate kapha because they are oily, cold, or predominantly sweet, sour, or salty.

★★Ghee is clarified butter; see recipe on page 32.

Vegetables:

Emphasize asparagus, cilantro, broccoli, cabbage, lettuce, alfalfa sprouts, mustard greens, chard, turnips, watercress, radishes, beets, carrots, pumpkin, celery, peas, green beans, chilies, lentils, lima beans, and soybeans. Eat moderate amounts of parsley, cauliflower, spinach, okra, squash, corn, seaweeds, chickpeas, split peas, tofu, and kidney and mung beans. Avoid cucumbers, avocado, and sweet potatoes.

Fruits:

Emphasize apples, cranberries, and dried fruits, and eat grapefruits, pomegranates, prunes, lemons, limes, and papayas in moderation. Avoid grapes, bananas, pineapple, oranges, pears, melons, plums, cherries, strawberries, mangoes, dates, and figs.

Grains:

Emphasize quinoa and barley; eat moderate amounts of corn, millet, buckwheat, rye, and basmati rice. Avoid oats, brown or white rice, and wheat.

Nuts, seeds, and oils:

Emphasize safflower, sunflower, grape-seed, and mustard oils; eat small quantities of coconut, pumpkin, sunflower, and sesame seeds, ghee★★, corn, peanut, and soy oils. Avoid walnuts, cashews, almonds, pine nuts, filberts, pecans, Brazil nuts and their oils, as well as butter, sesame, olive, and avocado oils.

Animal foods (nonvegetarians):

Use moderate amounts of buttermilk, skim or low-fat milk and low-fat cheese and yogurt, goat milk, and turkey and chicken; avoid all other animal and dairy products.

Sweeteners:

Use only clover honey, fruit juice concentrates, and Sucanat in moderation.

About Ghee (Clarified Butter)

Ayurveda considers *ghee,* or clarified butter, to be the most important lubricant you can ingest. Ghee is a light gourmet oil that increases enzyme production in your body. Therefore ghee helps you produce little engines that keep the whole body working at a much higher efficiency. I sometimes compare ghee with oil for a car's engine: A small amount goes a long way and is essential for the life of a car. The same is true of ghee and its relationship to your body. Ghee helps create ojas, improve sexual vitality, strengthen your nervous system, and build muscle. Ghee is used for cooking, particularly for sautéing vegetables; as a flavoring for vegetables or grains and cereals; as an ingredient in herbal medicines; and in skin care formulas. Because you use only a small amount, you needn't worry about increasing your risk of heart disease; butter contains only one gram of saturated fat per teaspoon, and a recent study found that the trans-fatty acids found in margarine is the most heart-unhealthy fat of all. The rich, silky, nutty flavor of ghee adds an incomparable flavor to foods and along with exotic spices, is what gives Indian foods their distinct taste and aroma.

You can buy a jar of ghee in Indian grocery stores, in some health food stores, and from the mail-order sources listed in the appendix of this book. But it's very simple to make at home:

1. Put one pound of unsalted organic butter in a stainless steel or heat-proof glass pan and place over medium heat.
2. Allow to melt and come to a boil; skim off the foam that forms on top. Lower the heat and allow the moisture to evaporate. The ghee will turn deep golden brown but should not burn.
3. Remove from heat, let cool, and strain into a storage jar. Store in your refrigerator, where it will keep indefinitely. Ghee will last up to two months without refrigeration.

EATING BEAUTIFULLY

If you gradually change your diet to conform to the dosha-appropriate guidelines, you'll be making great strides toward health and beauty. Eating

---

✳ THE TASTE OF HONEY ✳

If we remind you that honey comes from the nectar that bees delicately sip from flower blossoms, does it take a special place in your heart and dietary life? From the ancient Greeks to the people of the Hindus Valley honey was recognized not only for its sweet taste but also as an extraordinary life giving food. Honey is a natural high-energy food. It takes about ten minutes to get into the system and give the body a rush. Honey increases the absorption of calcium, is rich in vitamins and minerals, speeds the healing process, produces hemoglobin, and prevents anemia. It has antibiotic properties, and is an anti-viral, anti-inflammatory, anticarcinogenic, and antiallergenic. It works specifically on the skin, bones, and intestinal systems. Raw honey is high in enzymes and along with ghee stimulates the action that is needed for tissue synthesis. In Ayurveda, honey should never be used for cooking; but it may be added to foods after cooking. In Ayurveda honey is also categorized according to its doshic qualities. Vata types should limit themselves to orange blossom honey, pittas to wildflower honey, and kaphas to clover honey. If you have diabetes, please consult with your physician about the advisability of using honey.

Ayurvedically is automatically healthful because it provides a diet of balanced carbohydrate, protein, and fat that is also rich in nutrient-dense and fiber-full fresh fruits and vegetables and whole grains. But in Ayurveda, food is more than fuel to keep you going, more than a bunch of chemicals that supply essential vitamins and minerals. Wholesome food is a total experience that can nourish you emotionally as well as physically, creating a healthier, more beautiful you inside and out.

In Ayurveda, we are concerned not only with the chemical composition of the food you ingest, digest, and assimilate. The impact of what you taste, smell, see, hear, feel, and think is also important. In a sense, all you experience and take into your body-mind needs to be "nourishing" and "well digested" and distributed to all the parts of your body, mind and spirit. You'll learn more about food for the mind and spirit in the next chapter, but how well you nourish yourself also depends on the way in which the food you eat is raised, prepared, served, and consumed. In other words, "you are *how* you eat" too.

The following Ayurvedic recommendations, based on ancient observations and insights, are designed to help you cultivate beautiful eating habits so that the food you eat is nourishing in every way. Perhaps most profound is the concept that all foods and beverages are imprinted with a vital memory. Food "remembers" its whole life and, through its DNA, it also harbors remembrances of its ancestors' lives. Foods pass this rich store of knowledge to you when you eat them, providing a form of energy that connects them and you to other people and to the earth. Everyone, whether aware of it or not, longs to experience this link with the past and with Mother Earth. If your natural urge to have such positive emotional connections remain unfulfilled, you may try to get satisfaction in other ways; for example by eating too much food or eating beauty-sapping food or by becoming greedy and acquiring an excess of material things.

Choose Food Carefully

- Follow a vegetarian diet as closely as possible. This is not only better for your physical health, but has more beauty and grace psychologically and spiritually. Ayurveda minimizes heavy foods such as meat and cheese, which stress your digestive system.
- Milk, however, is considered to be one of the most important foods in Ayurveda; in India cows are sacred and treated with great respect, and the milk they give has powerful nourishing and healing qualities. If you drink milk or eat dairy products, we advise you to choose organic milk from cows raised under gentle conditions. Vegans and lactose-intolerant people may substitute organic soy, rice, or nut milks.
- Eat foods that have been grown or raised with care and attention. Food that is fresh, organically grown, and raised on small local farms, carries more positive, nourishing energy than food that is degraded and adulterated, raised with artificial chemicals, and impersonally grown on factory farms. Locally grown food is fresher and tastes better than conventional food, which travels on average 1,333 miles from farm to table. If you do eat meat, avoid commercial meat and poultry produced under stressful conditions for the animals and thus contain many negative memories that are passed on to you when you eat them.

- Shop in places you find esthetically pleasing and buy from pleasant people. Patronize quality health food stores and farmer's markets—or grow some of your own food so that you have a deeper connection with the earth from which your sustenance comes.

Cultivate Gracious Eating Habits

- Give eating the attention and respect it deserves. Sit down to eat, and don't rush. Avoid reading, watching TV, driving, or excited conversation while eating. Don't eat while you are upset; wait until you have calmed down. Focus on the food, chew it well, and take time to enjoy every mouthful so that you consciously and unconsciously take in the memory that food imparts, and your body-mind can assimilate the nutrients.
- Eat only when hungry, and don't overeat. Each meal should consist of about two and a half handfuls of food. After a meal you should be pleasantly satisfied, but not stuffed, and your stomach should contain one-third solid food and one-third liquid, with a third remaining empty so that there is space and energy for digestion.

Prepare and Serve Food Beautifully

- Put love and care into this essential activity. Prepare tasty and esthetically pleasing food. Pay attention to the details—the surroundings, the silverware, the dishes.
- Some foods are particularly beautiful, too—a plate of colorful vegetables or fruits, a nicely garnished serving dish or plate.
- It is nice when you are cooking for people you like and/or love and think of how they'll feel as you eat together. It is nice also to remember the people who taught you your recipes and to use some of their things (i.e., my grandmother's cast iron, my mother's knife, etc.).
- According to Ayurveda, the thoughts and emotions you have while handling food become part of your food. If you're angry or tense while preparing food, that's the energy you are taking in and feeding to other people. So, cook with positive emotions, such as love and kindness toward the food you are about to eat or share with others.
- When possible, use simple, nonmotorized hand tools to prepare

food—the more your own hands come into contact with food, the more opportunity for the food's energy to mix with yours, and the closer you feel to food and the earth from which it comes. Don't eat microwaved foods because according to Ayurveda they have had their life-force destroyed.

Other Eating Tips

- Most food should be eaten warm or hot—or at least room temperature—and usually cooked.
- Eat meals at about the same time every day, if possible, and eat your main meal at lunch. The timing of meals is believed to affect digestion, because your body goes through natural cycles of digestion and assimilation of food and elimination of waste. (More about this in Step 6.) This is especially important for calming excess vata. In addition, make sure you only eat food on an empty stomach; wait until your last meal has been digested, no matter what the clock says.
- Use small amounts of fats and oils. We recommend unhydrogenated, unrefined, cold-pressed oils; these are available at health food stores and Indian and Asian food stores. Ghee, or clarified butter, is also recommended in cooking and for flavoring. Oils are an important source of internal lubrication in Ayurveda. Vata, the driest dosha, has the least amount of lubrication and requires the most oil from food. Pittas have intense, hot body oils and need less oil from food. Kapha also have plenty of oils and need the least amount of outside oils.
- Sip warm or hot water before or during meals to aid digestion, but avoid icy or cold drinks before or with meals because they cool the digestive fire.
- Avoid refined sugar. Although some people require sweet foods, this doesn't mean fudge brownies. It means naturally sweet (fruits, grains, some vegetables such as carrots, sautéed onions, and sweet potatoes), which should still be eaten in moderation. Minimize refined sugar of all kinds; and use natural sweeteners in moderation, as appropriate to your dosha, such as honey, molasses, or Sucanat. Minimize alcohol and coffee in general and especially with meals. They deplete your body of needed nutrients, accelerate aging, form free radicals, overburden your system, and add toxins.

- After eating, take a short, gentle walk and never sleep right after eating—make sure you leave a few hours in between.
- Eat foods that work together in combination. **Avoid** the following combinations because when eaten together these foods create poor digestion, malabsorption, and clogging of the channels:

Milk or yogurt . . . with sour fruits, fish, potatoes, eggplant, or tomatoes

Melons . . . with any other food

Bananas . . . with milk, corn, starches, or radishes

Meat . . . with milk, yogurt, or eggs

Cheese . . . with yogurt, eggs, or mango

Bread . . . with milk

Eggs . . . with milk, yogurt, or starchy food

Starches . . . with yogurt, milk, dates, or persimmons

Cucumbers . . . with mango, lemon, potato, eggplant, or tomato

ABOUT HERBS AND SPICES

Ayurveda has its own unique view of herbs and spices and how they work. Herbs are thought of, first of all, as a kind of concentrated food. So, although herbs affect the body through several discrete mechanisms—they contain vitamins, minerals, hormones, and chemicals that act as stimulants and relaxants, and so on—Ayurveda traditionally classifies them according to their taste and how they affect the three doshas.

In Ayurveda, herbs and spices are consumed every day as flavorful teas and in cooked food dishes. In addition to shaping your diet according to Ayurvedic food guidelines, you can choose dosha-appropriate herbs and spices and integrate them into your daily eating pattern. These potent packets of nourishment work synergistically with food to help balance your doshas, boost energy, focus your mind, and rejuvenate all the tissues and organs of your body.

Generally, herbs and spices are used in powdered form. You can buy most of the herbs we recommend at most health food stores, farmer's markets, and many food markets. Others are sold at Indian grocery stores and through the mail by sources listed in the "Mail Order Suppliers" section of this book. Make sure your herbs are fresh when you buy them and store them in a dark, dry place for up to one year (mark the expiration date on the container.)

Cooking with Herbs and Spices

Herbs and spices add flavor and zip to your meals while balancing the doshas. Experiment with the herbs and spices listed below, or use one of the Ayurvedic cookbooks (see the "Further Reading" section of this book), which will teach you how to prepare delicious, flavorful foods that taste good and are good for you. Once again, these herbs are chosen on the basis of their effects on the doshas. To calm vata, emphasize sweet, sour, and salty herbs, spices, and flavorings; to cool pitta, emphasize herbs and spices that are sweet, bitter, and astringent; to stimulate kapha, emphasize herbs and spices that are pungent, bitter, and astringent.

VATA—CALMING HERBS AND SPICES
Fennel, oregano, sage, tarragon, thyme, cinnamon, basil, cardamom, coriander, and cumin

PITTA—COOLING HERBS AND SPICES
Fresh cilantro, fresh ginger, cumin, coriander, fennel, chamomile, turmeric, mint, cinnamon, cardamom, and nutmeg

KAPHA—STIMULATING HERBS AND SPICES
Black pepper, cayenne, garlic, mustard, fresh ginger, cinnamon, cloves, cardamom, turmeric, coriander, fresh cilantro, and cumin

Spiced Herbal Teas

Spiced herbal teas are a gentle yet effective way to use herbs and spices every day. The easiest way is to buy commercially prepared tea bags, available at health food stores and from "Mail-Order Suppliers" (see page 190). Yogi Tea, available at some health food stores, is an all-purpose blend beneficial for all doshas. There are also commercially available herbal blends labeled Vata-Pacifying, Pitta-Pacifying, or Kapha-Pacifying, designed for specific doshas. Alternatively, you can make your own yogi, vata, pitta, and kapha teas, using the recipes provided below.

Make a pot of tea in the morning; have one cup at breakfast, instead of coffee, black tea, or your usual caffeine and/or sugar-laden beverage. Drink the rest throughout the day (take some in a thermos to work). You can experiment with the proportions of herbs and spices to get a blend that most pleases your palate; just aim to use one teaspoon total per brewed cup of tea.

Yogi Tea

This is a tri-doshic tea, good for general balancing of all three doshas. Boil 8 cups of water in a stainless steel saucepan. Add:

2 tsp. fresh grated ginger
4 whole cardamom seeds, slightly crushed
1 whole cinnamon stick, slightly crushed
8 whole cloves

Boil for twenty minutes. Strain and drink warm or cooled to room temperature, and add sweetener and milk, if desired.

Vata-Balancing Tea

This tea calms vata, which goes out of balance by becoming aggravated. Boil 4 cups of water in a stainless steel saucepan. Reduce heat and stir in:

2 tsp. fresh grated ginger
1 tsp. whole cardamom seeds, slightly crushed
2 whole cinnamon sticks, slightly crushed
⅛ tsp. saffron

Let simmer, covered, for 10 minutes. Remove from heat and let steep 5 more minutes. To serve, strain and add fresh boiled milk and honey, if desired. This makes about 3½ cups of tea. You may reheat it or drink it room temperature.

· · · · · · PITTA-BALANCING TEA · · · · · ·

Chamomile or mint tea are simple easy teas to brew for soothing pitta. The following combination more forcefully cools and strengthens pitta, which goes out of balance by becoming overheated. Boil 4 cups of water in a stainless steel saucepan. Remove pan from heat and stir in:

2 tsp. fresh grated ginger
1 tsp. whole cardamom seeds, slightly crushed
1½ tsp. spearmint or other mint
2 whole cinnamon sticks, slightly crushed

Cover the tea and let it steep for at least 10 minutes. To serve, strain, squeezing out as much of the liquid as you can; add maple syrup, if desired. This makes about 3½ cups of strong tea; dilute with two cups of water if it seems too strong for you. Sip hot or cool as desired.

· · · · · · KAPHA-BALANCING TEA · · · · ·

This stimulating beverage serves to invigorate kapha, which tends to become more sluggish when out of balance, mentally and physically. Boil 4 cups of water in a stainless steel saucepan. Reduce heat and stir in:

1 tsp. whole cardamom seeds, slightly crushed
1 tsp. whole cloves
⅛ tsp. black pepper
1 T. peeled and chopped fresh gingerroot

Let simmer, covered, for at least 10 minutes. To serve, strain and add honey to sweeten if desired. This makes about 3½ cups.

Now that you've learned how to nourish your body, you're ready to go to the next step: nourishing the invisible part of your self—your mind and spirit. In Ayurveda, the intangible self is not separate from the tangible self, so that what you've learned in this chapter will contribute to a beautiful inner you, and what you learn in the next chapter will support your outer beauty as well.

STEP 3

Nourishing Your Mind and Spirit

*M*ANY WOMEN COME INTO MY OFFICE WHO ARE DOING everything right—eating nourishing food appropriate to their doshas, exercising, taking vitamin supplements, and possibly practicing some form of "stress management"—yet they do not look or feel their best. Instead of brimming with health and joy and beauty, they radiate negative energy, feel down on life, and wear their discontent on their faces. They have problems with their skin, complexion, weight, and energy level. They are neglecting their minds and spirits, and that's why Step 3 in our program involves embracing and integrating practices that cultivate inner beauty into your life.

Most people acknowledge that mental and emotional stress is a beauty killer—but Ayurveda goes beyond this simple observation. It concerns itself not just with what to avoid, in other words, how to reduce stress, but also what to seek out. As is the case with food and herbs, you can nourish yourself with beautiful, positive, pleasurable thoughts, feelings, and experiences. This creates ojas—the health- and beauty-building juice of life. Or you can starve yourself even while clogging up your system with harmful versions of these intangible aspects of existence. This psychic malnutrition creates an empty longing as well as ama—the accumulation of toxins—just as surely as poor eating creates them.

In this chapter, we show you how Ayurvedic practices can help you reach your innermost self. We give you tools to help you radiate contentment—the most profound beauty there is. We begin by discussing what stress is and then provide stress-relieving, bliss-creating techniques—breathing and relaxation exercises and meditation—to prevent the everyday wear and tear that can ruin your health and your appearance. Next, you'll find a primer on yoga and a basic set of yoga positions to help you integrate body, mind, and spirit and feel more centered, grounded, strong, and flexible physically, mentally, and emotionally. We also provide exercise guidelines for each dosha to help you individualize your fitness program. Finally, we introduce you to Five-Senses Therapy—using touch, taste, sight, sound, and aromas—to wake up all your senses and enliven your mind and spirit. These discussions are necessarily brief; for more detail and information, please refer to our earlier book, *Ayurveda: The A–Z Guide to Healing Techniques from Ancient India.*

HOW STRESS SAPS BEAUTY

Who hasn't made the connection between stress, worry, and skin problems such as pimples and signs of premature aging, wrinkles, and facial lines? Who hasn't heard about or experienced "anxious overeating" leading to overweight, or stress-induced loss of appetite leading to painful thinness? In addition to these obvious beauty killers, it's been well documented that prolonged stress wreaks all sorts of health havoc: it can contribute to fatigue, diabetes, hypertension, ulcers, loss of libido, reduced resistance to disease, irregular menstrual periods, reduced fertility, and difficult menopause. Stress is rampant in the modern world: in 1993, the U.S. Public Health Survey estimated that 70 to 80 percent of Americans who visit physicians suffer from a stress-related disorder.

What Is Stress?

In Ayurveda, the mind (consciousness) and the body (physical matter) not only influence each other—they *are* each other. Together, they form the body-mind. There can be no physical health or physical attractiveness without mental health. It should come as no surprise, then, that in Ayurveda, thoughts or feelings are just as important as the physical body.

Biologically, you are hard-wired to respond to threatening situations.

When you perceive something to be stressful, an internal alarm goes off, triggering a cascade of chemical secretions and physiological changes that has been called a "fight or flight" response. Your mind and body go into red alert, the better to fight for your life or to get away from the danger as fast as possible. Then once the danger is over, you can relax, and everything goes back to normal—but a new, stronger normal fed by your experience with past hardships.

For centuries, Ayurveda has recognized stress as the ebb and flow of the physiology's response to life. Such painful, negative emotions as fear, anger, and grief aren't necessarily harmful. These are all good, natural human emotions under certain conditions. When you are healthy, you can "digest" and metabolize stress and painful negative feelings. You even benefit from them because you actually convert them to useful energy that helps you grow and develop.

However, there is such a thing as too much stress. In that case, you're always at least slightly on hyperalert—with some part of your system revved up and others tamped down. Such a tired or hysterical system cannot manage to ride the waves of your physiology. Your system produces ama (undigested energy that turns toxic), which accumulates and clogs the system. A vicious cycle ensues: The more stress you experience, the less able you are to cope with it, the less you are able to recover from it, and the less you are able to deal with new stressors. There's all flow and no ebb—waves crashing into one another, creating biochemical chaos. This chemistry of negativity eventually harms tissues and is a prescription for disaster—ulcers, heart problems, skin rashes, insomnia, bags and circles under the eyes, worry lines, and a lifeless complexion.

Mindfulness

You can break the cycle of stress and negative thoughts through the practice of self-knowledge and daily observation that is sometimes called "mindfulness." The challenge is to unlearn your habitual responses that are not working. The first step is to realize that the way you respond to any situation depends in part on your own unique fears and your conditioning—what has happened to you in the past and how you have managed to cope. The next step is to recognize them and acknowledge them. This takes self-observation and contemplation, the ability to know yourself, to be open and honest about yourself and your beliefs and behaviors, to know who you are without judging. Studying the doshas is the preliminary tool. This teaches you about your essential nature, your innate strengths and weaknesses—and it also shines a light on your true potential.

When you can live mindfully, something miraculous happens—you open the door to entirely new possibilities, new ways of perceiving stressful situations. For example, everyone gets stuck in traffic at some time. But only you can determine if you will fume and grit your teeth and give in to road rage. Everyone loses someone dear to them at some point, but only you can decide if you will get stuck and mourn the loss forever, or let the heavy mantle of bitterness or guilt ruin your chance of enjoying your own life.

Realize that this kind of work is difficult to do on your own. To help you find your own path of self-exploration and growth, seek counseling, spiritual teachers, support groups, friends, books, the arts, philosophy. Changing your ways can be frightening, and it's not easy. But the rewards are great. In giving up your old ways of looking at things and reacting to them, you gain control and power. You are not the helpless, impotent victim, buffeted this way and that by the big and little vagaries of life. How you react to any situation is really up to you. To put the principle of mindfulness to work for you:

- *Vata types* tend to be quick and light in your thoughts; but when out of balance, their thoughts turn chaotic. Vatas must be mindful of their thinking process and observe their thoughts go by so that they become conscious of their pattern.
- *Pitta types* are characteristically discriminating; this is a gift, but they can get caught up in a web of being overly judgmental. Pittas must contemplate their judgments.
- *Kapha types* are prized for their slow, steady, thought process. But when out of balance, thinking can become stuck and stagnant, so kaphas need to be mindful of their thoughts and ask whether they are obsessing about the same thought again and again.

Create Your Own Release Valve

In addition to mindfulness, another way to improve your emotional digestion is to create a release valve with stress-reducing activities. Choose the technique that is right for you from the following traditional Ayurvedic techniques that we have brought up to date. We hope you'll choose more than one, because they have quite different characteristics and demand different time commitments. These breathing exercises, muscle relaxation techniques, and meditations are easy, efficient, and inexpensive. They fit into modern life quite easily. Everyone can find time to breathe in a particular way for five minutes twice a day or to close the eyes and repeat a prayer or a mantra for twenty minutes every day.

BREATHING PRACTICES (*PRANAYAMA*)

Breathing exercises are called pranayama (PRAH-nah-YAH-mah). They are a part of the discipline of yoga (see below) and are said to help balance consciousness, improve creativity, allow us to feel joy, bliss, peace, and love. Ayurveda recommends that special attention be paid to breathing because *prana*, the vital life-force, enters the body with each breath.

Traditionally, these exercises are done while sitting comfortably cross-legged on the floor; if you want to use this position, you should elevate your sitting bones with one or two large folded towels or a meditation cushion. Loose-fitting, comfortable clothes and dark, quiet surroundings also help but are not required. You can do these breathing practices anywhere, any time you need to "take five," during a yoga practice, or as a prelude to meditation. Five minutes at your desk twice during an eight-hour shift will have an immediate effect on increasing energy and clarity.

Abdominal Breathing

This simple technique teaches you to fill your entire lungs with air, massaging your internal organs, and reducing anxiety, depression, nervousness, muscle tension, and fatigue. It may also pave the way for your entering the "alpha state," in which the mind is exceptionally calm and clear.

1. To begin, sit or lie down in a comfortable position. Rest one hand over your abdomen and one on your upper chest. Take a few slow

breaths and notice where your breath goes—does your chest rise and fall but not your abdomen? Or does your abdomen move alone?

2. Next, breathe in slowly through your nose, attempting to fill your abdomen first, by lowering your diaphragm. This may take several tries—imagine your abdomen is a balloon.
3. Once your abdomen is filled, keep inhaling and fill your chest, allowing it to rise.
4. Exhale slowly through your mouth, first emptying your chest and then your abdomen.
5. Repeat the inhalation and exhalation, trying to slow the breath even more. This should feel like a wave of air, rhythmically entering and leaving your body.

Alternate Nostril Breathing

The purpose of alternating nostrils as instructed below is to stabilize vata. To cool and balance pitta, breathe in only through the left nostril and breathe out through the right; to heat and stimulate kapha, inhale through the right nostril only and exhale through the left. For best results, use abdominal breathing, described above, for the inhalations and exhalations.

1. Using your right hand, place your thumb next to your right nostril and your middle finger next to your left nostril. Gently but firmly close off your right nostril with your thumb. Inhale through your left nostril, bringing your awareness to your heart.
2. Release your right nostril and close off your left nostril with your middle finger, exhaling through your right nostril.
3. Keeping your left nostril closed, inhale through your right nostril.
4. Close off your right nostril and inhale through your left nostril.
5. Repeat this breathing pattern twelve times.

PROGRESSIVE MUSCLE RELAXATION

You can also use abdominal breathing during this technique, which involves alternately tensing and then relaxing each muscle group of your

---

❋ EYE PILLOWS TO QUIET YOUR MIND ❋

Eye pillows are a delicious way to aid relaxation. Placing one of these lavender-scented, pleasantly weighted flaxseed-filled items over your eyes shuts out distracting light, quiets the eyes, and gently massages tired eye muscles. The scent of lavender is known for its ability to relax you. Available at many New Age shops and through Living Arts by mail (see "Mail-Order Suppliers" appendix, page 190); they are also easy to make. Simply cut two 4"×8" pieces of silk, sew together around three sides, fill loosely with flaxseed and dried lavender, and stitch up the fourth side.

---

body. You may want to use a scented eye pillow (see "Eye Pillows to Quiet Your Mind," above) to induce deeper relaxation. Breathe slowly, deeply, and rhythmically throughout, inhaling during a contraction and forcefully exhaling as you let go.

To do the practice, lie down on a comfortable surface, close your eyes, and take a few deep, slow breaths. Direct your attention to your right leg. Stretch it away from your body, pointing your foot hard; hold until it begins to tremble slightly, and then let go and allow it to relax completely. Repeat with the left leg. Next, move your attention to your right arm, stretch it, and then let it go limp, as you did with your leg. Clench your hand into a tight fist; hold and then release. Stretch the fingers out straight; hold and then release. Proceed to alternately contract and then relax the muscles of your buttocks, stomach muscles, back muscles, shoulders, and face. After taking a few deep, slow breaths, repeat the exercise. Then just lie still for ten minutes or so, allowing your mind to let go of whatever is bothering you.

MEDITATION

Mindfulness helps you alter the way you perceive stress, and breathing and relaxation techniques help release stressful feelings, but they are not the whole picture. These techniques work best if they take place in an internal

---

❋ BENEFITS OF MEDITATION: IT'S NOT ALL IN YOUR MIND ❋

Over the years, thousands of meditators have been studied to assess the benefits of the practice. The results are astounding. Meditating is deeply relaxing and rejuvenating; it reduces blood levels of stress hormones, which are associated with poor health and aging. It lowers or normalizes blood pressure, pulse rate, and abnormally high cholesterol levels. It enhances immune system response and increases alpha brain-wave activity, which is present during times of creativity and relaxation. In fact, some long-term meditators have been found to be five to twelve years younger biologically than they are chronologically, as indicated by their blood pressure, visual acuity, and hearing. New research shows that meditators have up to nearly 50 percent higher levels of a hormone called DHEA. Low levels of DHEA are considered to be a marker for exposure to chronic stress and a mirror for aging.

---

landscape that is balanced, open, fertile, and receptive. Creating that landscape is a job for meditation.

Meditation is a tool to help you develop a restful alertness and inner peace. Many people find that with regular meditation, they experience a profound shift in their inner lives. This in turn can also positively affect physical health, aging, and appearance.

How to Meditate

Meditation is a different experience for each person, and each session is different as well. The following exercise will help you get a glimpse of what meditation feels like. Before beginning, choose a word or phrase to bring your attention to, such as the word "Om" or the ancient Sanskrit mantra *Ham Sah*, meaning "I am that." Most people start out meditating for twenty minutes and work up to thirty or forty-five minutes. You can easily lose track of time in deep relaxation, so you may need to set a timer or stopwatch if you don't have unlimited time.

Situate yourself in a quiet place where you won't be disturbed by the phone or other people. If possible, create a special place of beauty and repose for your practice, no matter how modest. Include a plant, a vase of fresh flowers, a painting, candles, incense—anything that helps you set apart this place, this quiet time for yourself. It is said that if you meditate in the same place regularly, you influence the energy present in the room, creating a peaceful oasis that your consciousness recognizes from the moment you enter it. This sets the stage for a more powerful, effortless meditation that is enhanced each time you practice. Aim to meditate once a day at the same time; twice if possible. The best times are sunrise and sunset.

1. Sit in a comfortable position that you can hold for at least twenty minutes. A traditional posture is to sit cross-legged on the floor, sitting bones elevated by a meditation cushion (one or more folded towels can substitute).
2. Close your eyes; you may prepare yourself by doing the abdominal breathing exercise described above.
3. Let your eyes roll upward and focus on the spot on your forehead between your eyes, keeping all facial muscles as relaxed as possible. Repeat the focus word(s) silently; as you do so, thoughts will enter your head. Just let them drift by as you breathe deeply and rhythmically. You can time your words or phrases with your breath, keeping the inhale broad, deep, and easy and the exhale silent and effortless.
4. When your time is up, remain seated for a minute or two with your eyes closed, and then open them. Slowly begin to move your body, and ease yourself back into waking consciousness.

YOGA

The practice of yoga is a kind of moving meditation; it may also incorporate mental exercises. The word *yoga* is derived from the Sanskrit word *yug*, which means "to yoke or harness." Traditionally, this is interpreted as "joining" the consciousness of an individual with the universal consciousness. It has also come to mean the union between the mind and body.

In yoga, the breath is an intrinsic part of the practice because it is thought that prana, the vital life-force, enters the body with each breath. There are many schools of yoga, but *hatha* (HA-tha) *yoga* is the form most commonly practiced in Western countries. This form emphasizes physical postures or "poses," called *asanas* (AH-sah-nahs), that you enter and hold for several breaths. *Iyengar* (eye-EN-gar) *yoga*, which emphasis correct alignment and utilizes props to help you achieve this, is one popular school of yoga. *Astanga* (ah-STENG-ah) is another school that is gaining in popularity in the United States, where it is also called power yoga. In this form, you flow through the poses nonstop in a beautiful display of strength, grace, and fluidity. Every pose is connected to the next, giving it the feel of a dance rather than the static stop-and-go rhythm you may be familiar with. Iyengar and astanga yoga can be quite strenuous and intense, creating a surprising amount of heat in your body. This causes you to perspire, eliminating toxins and rejuvenating the entire system; it also allows you to stretch more deeply into each pose.

Yoga works on the inside and the outside simultaneously. As a long-time yoga practitioner says, "Yoga has not only strengthened and opened up my body; it has also loosened, strengthened, and opened up my heart and soul." The calmness achieved during the practice carries over into the rest of your life. I have noticed that yoga students and teachers tend to look and act younger than their chronological years. When done for a period of time, yoga helps balance your nervous, endocrine, reproductive, and circulatory systems and your digestive tract. It relieves tension and pain in your joints and builds strength, flexibility, balance, and grace; it allows you to avoid or counteract the undesirable effects of other activities such as tight, short muscles, limited range of motion, and misalignment.

You can learn yoga from books and videotapes, but it's best to participate in yoga classes (or get individual instruction), especially if you're new to the practice. Classes and private lessons are available in health clubs, fitness centers, dance centers, yoga centers, and community centers. As with any exercise program, check with your doctor before beginning yoga.

Sun Salutation Sequence (Surya Namaskar)

Sun Salutation is a flowing, full-body exercise that is carefully designed to work all the major muscle groups and joints and massage your internal organs. This sequence of poses is traditionally performed in the early morning, as the sun rises. During the sequence, you stretch up and down, forward and back. You support your body weight with your arms, and with your legs. You expand and contract the front and back of your body. Simple though it is, if you perform this sequence every day with joy and love and understanding, you will experience subtle differences in your consciousness as well as dramatic differences in the way your body feels, looks, and moves.

We recommend that you perform the entire Sun Salutation sequence at least five times each morning. Begin slowly, with fewer repetitions, if you are new to yoga or physical activity. Gradually build up to five sequences, and rest when you need to, preferably in the Child's Pose shown on page 58. Vata types should continue to do these movements slowly; pittas should move at a moderate pace; and kaphas should aim to do them rapidly.

As you practice yoga, coordinate your breathing with the movements: inhale during movements that stretch the spine and open the body; exhale during movements that involve bending or folding of the spine or limbs. Imagine each breath as an extension of the pose, and keep your movements fluid and precise as you work to open up and extend your entire spine in each position. Be conscious of your hands and feet as the foundation of each pose; imagine they are lotus blossoms, and spread your fingers and toes as if they were lotus petals. As you flow through the sequence, imagine you are standing high on a hilltop in India, with the sun breaking over the distant mountains, the sky exploding in the brilliant colors of dawn. As the birds greet the day, they chirp and swoop for joy at the gift of existence. As you raise your arms, extend your legs, and feel your lungs expanding and contracting, you also feel the joy of new beginnings and all of life coursing through your body.

Yoga is best performed on an empty stomach, in bare feet, while wearing loose or stretchy clothing, on a non-skid surface. Set the mood with a bouquet of flowers or a living plant on which you can focus your gaze, and turn off the phone ringer.

When you have completed the sequence, rest in the Child's Pose until your breathing comes back to normal. You may also use this position to rest between sets if you need to. Then lie on your back with legs extended, arms at a 45-degree angle from your sides and relax with your eyes closed for a few minutes.

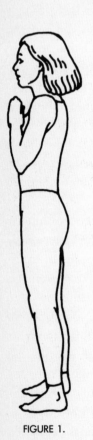

FIGURE 1.

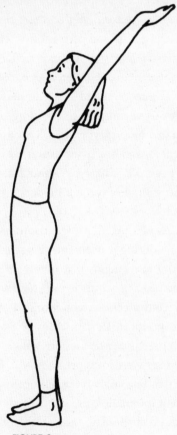

FIGURE 2.

PRAYER POSE

(*Pranamasana*): Stand tall, feet hip-width apart and parallel. Place your palms together, prayer position, midchest. Take a few moments to become centered and focused.

RAISED ARMS POSE

(*Hasta Uttanasana*). Inhale as you stretch and sweep your arms out to the side and then overhead. Stretch your breastbone up to the sky and your tailbone down to the earth, elongating your spine. You may arch your upper back slightly, but avoid arching the lower back or raising the shoulders.

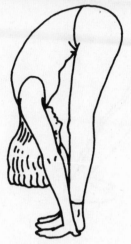

FIGURE 3.

STANDING FORWARD BEND

(*Uttanasana*). Exhale as you bend over from the hips, sweeping your arms out to the side and placing your palms flat on the floor, one on each side of your feet. Ideally, your knees should be straight, but not locked; you may need to bend them at first to get your palms flat to the floor.

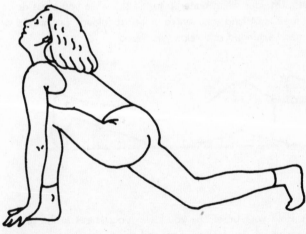

FIGURE 4.

WARRIOR POSE

(*Virabhadrasana*). Inhale as you extend your left leg back in a lunge position. Position your right leg so that it makes a right angle, keeping your calf perpendicular to the floor and your foot flat. You may drop your left knee to the ground or keep it straight. Remember to keep lengthening your spine and avoid hunching your shoulders or squeezing your neck.

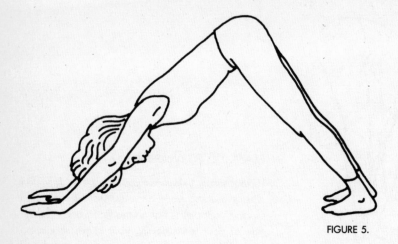

FIGURE 5.

DOWNWARD DOG POSE

(*Adhomukha Shvanasana*). Exhale, bringing your right leg back to meet the left leg, feet hip-width apart. Lift your sitting bone up to the sky while you press down with your hands and feet, stretching your entire spine, shoulders, and backs of your legs. Keep your neck extended and relax your head.

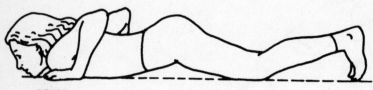

FIGURE 6.

EIGHT LIMBS POSE

(*Ashtanganamaskara*). Hold your breath as you lower your knees to the ground and then bend your arms as you lower your chest and chin to the floor. Keep your toes curled under and your buttocks raised off the floor; the "eight limbs" are your feet, knees, hands, chest, and chin.

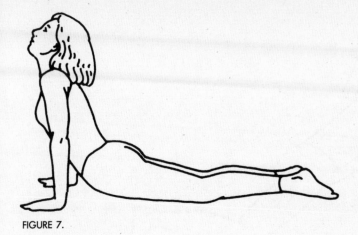

FIGURE 7.

COBRA POSE

(*Bhujangasana*). Inhale as you press down with your hands and begin to straighten your arms as you scoop your chest forward and up. Your elbows should remain close to your body and only arch your lower back as far as it can comfortably go. Move your breastbone up and out, and make sure to widen and drop your shoulders down away from your neck, rather than scrunch your neck and shoulders together. You may need to keep your elbows bent at first to avoid pinching your lower back.

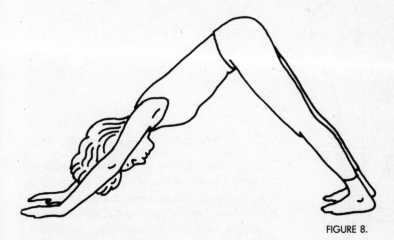

FIGURE 8.

DOWNWARD DOG POSE

(*Adhomukha Shvanasana*). Exhale as you repeat Pose 5, trying to lengthen your spine even more as your press your hands and the balls of your feet into the floor, stretching your heels down.

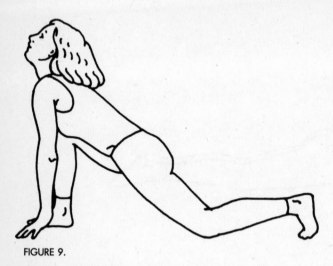

FIGURE 9.

WARRIOR POSE

(*Virabhadrasana*). Inhale as you repeat Pose #4, bringing the left leg forward so your foot is flat between your hands.

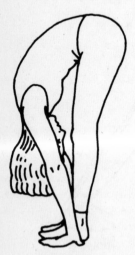

FIGURE 10.

STANDING FORWARD BEND

(*Uttanasana*). Exhale as you step forward with the right foot and repeat Pose 3. Be careful not to round your upper back; the object is not to touch your head to your knee or to get your legs straight; rather it is to extend and lengthen the spine out and over from the hips, not the waist.

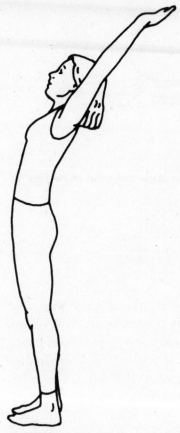

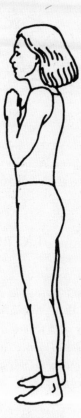

FIGURE 11.

FIGURE 12.

RAISED ARMS POSE

(*Hasta Uttanasana*). Inhale deeply as you repeat Pose 2.

PRAYER POSE

(*Pranamasna*): Exhale as you bring your arms back to Pose 1. Take a few resting breaths before you repeat the set of twelve poses.

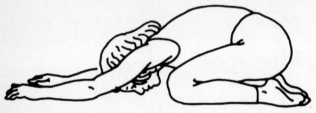

FIGURE 13.

CHILD'S POSE.

Big toes touching, knees apart, sit back on your heels and bend at the hips, extending your arms in front of you.

EXERCISE GUIDELINES

What is exercise doing in a chapter on mind and spirit? Study after study confirms that physical activity reduces tension, improves sleep, improves memory and reaction time, lessens depression and elevates mood, and boosts self-confidence and self-esteem. Exercise takes your mind off your troubles, burns off adrenaline, and stimulates the secretion of endorphins and serotonin, those feel-good neurochemicals. Not surprisingly, it can also improve your sex life.

Of course, exercise has physical benefits too: it has been shown to improve lung function, burn fat, increase stamina, lower blood pressure, improve resistance to disease and reduce risk of coronary heart disease, stroke, osteoporosis, diabetes and possibly many types of cancer. Experiments have shown that physical activity, along with a diet rich in vitamins A, C, and E, may help keep skin more youthful, because the skin continues to produce *sebum*, the body's natural lubricant and moisturizer.

In Ayurveda, exercise is recognized as good preventive medicine and all-around beauty treatment because it also enables more prana to reach the tissues by cleaning and clearing all channels, which promotes circulation, supplies nutrients, and encourages excretion of wastes.

The best news is that recent studies suggest that moderate exercise can be beneficial. Aim for a total of thirty minutes every day of moderate intensity. And short periods of everyday activities and chores such as raking

leaves, walking, dancing, gardening, and playing with the kids can accumulate and be as beneficial as an equivalent amount of time spent "working
out." Walking, it turns out, may be the best, most versatile, convenient,
and easiest way to be physically active. It is a wonderful complement to
yoga practice.

Ayurveda has long advocated a moderate approach to exercise. It warns
you not to overdo it, because overexertion could shorten life span and lower
resistance to disease. In Ayurveda, the rule of thumb is to avoid spending
more than half your energy on exercise; so if an hour of running exhausts
you, don't run for more than a half hour at a time. The exertion level
should be just enough to cause you to sweat on your forehead, under your
arms, and along your spinal column—this is the level at which activity
stimulates agni, relaxes you and helps you sleep. Sweating reduces toxins,
burns fat, and elevates mood by producing endorphins. But beware of becoming addicted to endorphins (your body's natural morphine), a habit that
is especially common in vata types.

Ayurveda also teaches that exercise is a highly individual matter. Use
your dosha as a guide to type, duration, and intensity of activity:

- *Vata types*: When vata predominates, you tend to prefer the most
vigorous workouts, but you also get too exhausted if you exercise too
strenuously for too long. Since vata types are prone to joint problems,
emphasize low-impact activities. You do well with slow low-intensity
rhythmic exercises such as medium-paced walking, yoga, dancing,
swimming, easy low-impact aerobics, and Tai Chi. Be sure to drink
plenty of water before, during, and after activity and to rest afterward.
- *Pitta types*: If your prakruti is dominated by pitta, the fiery dosha, you
tend to have an athletic body and an intense, competitive, aggressive
nature. You do well with competitive sports and steady, medium-
intensity exercises such as aerobic and jazz dance, ballet, non-contact
martial arts, doubles tennis and team sports, adventurous, rugged
outdoor activities such as skiing, hiking, hang gliding, canoeing,
white-water rafting, and cooling activities such as swimming. Remember, exercise can be intense and competitive, but not at the
expense of being fun. Guard against becoming overheated or over-
exercised, which makes you irritable and exhausted, and be sure to
rest adequately between activities.

• *Kapha types*: If you are mostly kapha, the lethargic dosha, you need lengthy, vigorous, stimulating workouts to control weight, boost circulation and digestion, and stimulate your mind. Top picks are aerobic dance, jogging and running, basketball, and weight training five or six times a week. But since you are the most resistant to physical activity, anything is better than nothing, so indulge in whatever is enjoyable and available—ballroom dancing, walking the dog, bowling, and anything that gets you moving.

FIVE-SENSES THERAPY: KEEPING ALL THE DOORS OPEN

The world is such a beautiful place, filled with natural and human-made things to see, taste, feel, smell, and hear: sunsets, trees, paintings, music, the sweet song of a bird, a lover's caress, a baby's tiny fingers wrapping around your finger, home-cooked meals, just-picked berries, night-blooming jasmine, a Bach partita. Yet we often limit our exposure to such pleasures or accept intrusive, unpleasant sensations: windowless, airless rooms, concrete landscapes, the din and stench of traffic, McFood, a cold, hard plastic chair to rest our weary bones. With all this gracelessness how can we hope to be beautiful ourselves? Seeing beauty in our surroundings, in others, and in ourselves is a deeply satisfying experience. Computer experts say, "Garbage in, garbage out." Andrew Weil, in *Spontaneous Healing* says, "Beauty in any form has a salutary effect on spirit." Ayurveda says, essentially, "Beauty in, beauty out."

According to Ayurveda, your five senses—sight, taste, touch, smell, and hearing—are the doorways to your inner being. Five-Senses Therapy, which I use in my clinical practice to restore and maintain balance to the doshas, involves simple practices that are among the most pleasurable and effective techniques in Ayurveda. I often begin treating my patients with Five-Senses Therapy because it is so easy and pleasurable to use and because of its speedy effect. There's growing evidence that feeling good is good for you. Pleasurable feelings, it seems, are the antidote to negative stress. Pleasure creates endorphins, the chemicals that reduce the effects of stress and

---

❀ MASSAGE IN INDIA ❀

In India, massage is a natural part of daily life. It's common for entire families to massage each other once a week. Infants are massaged every day from the day they are born to age three and weekly after that. By age six, children are massaging their elders, and pregnant women are massaged daily during pregnancy and for over a month after giving birth. Sensual massage with aphrodisiac oils is advised in treatises on sexology.

---

create the feeling of bliss, or ojas in Sanskrit. What could be more beauty-enhancing than that?

Touch: Massage Therapy and More

Massage is an essential component of our program because skin is nerve rich and intimately connected with the vata dosha, the one that governs the nervous system. Because of vata's dry, electrical nature, it is essential to lubricate the skin and mucus membranes with oils to insulate the electrical nerve impulses. During Ayurvedic massage, oils are used that penetrate the skin and the entire nervous system, nourishing the beauty within and bringing radiant beauty to the skin surface.

But there's much more to the sense of touch than massage. We live in an increasing "virtual" world, one step removed from the real thing—from electronic shopping to indoor treadmill workouts. Each inch of your skin contains 9,000 nerve endings, and they are hungry for a more varied tactile life. If you spend most of your time with fingertips pressing the plastic keys on a keyboard, it's time to get back in touch and put more variety in your tactile experience. Here are a few ideas to get you started:

- Make bread and knead the dough by hand—you'll be surprised how satisfying this can be, and you have the added plus of satisfying your taste buds later on.
- Dig in the garden—even if you are an urbanite, you can have a few flower pots on a windowsill to bring the joy of nurturing to your day.
- Take barefoot walks on the beach or on soft grass.

- Work with clay or another sculpture material.
- Find a dog or cat to pet regularly, and enjoy the soft luxuriousness of its fur, perhaps by volunteering at an animal shelter.
- Do you touch the significant people in your life often enough? Do they touch you? Make an effort to have greater physical contact—a pat on the arm, a reassuring touch on the shoulder—when appropriate.
- Give yourself an oil massage. With every stroke you are letting your body and mind know that you care enough to perform this marvelous, loving ritual. Instructions for self-massage appear in the chapter devoted to Step 5.
- Massage is also soothing and calming for the person who gives it. So part of your beauty program could be massaging your mate, parent, sibling, or other relative or close friend. You might begin informally, with a simple back rub, using your own intuition, and relying on feedback to help you learn and improve your technique.
- Get a professional massage. Ayurveda massage emphasizes 108 specific points, called *marmas* (MAR-mahs), that are extremely sensitive and crucial for maintaining balanced doshas. Similar to acupuncture points, marma points are believed to be where the physical body meets the mind.

Taste: Spice Therapy

Taste is of profound importance in the way Ayurveda understands the human body-mind, as we explained in Step 2. There are nine thousand taste buds, and when stimulated, they trigger nerve impulses to special taste centers in the brain's cortex and thalamus. If you don't have all six tastes, or *rasas* (RAH-sahs), every day, your brain is being deprived of nourishing stimulation. There are several easy ways to wake up your taste buds and nourish your mind and spirit:

- If you continually favor the same limited group of foods, use the food lists in Step 2 (pages 28–31) to get out of your food rut.
- Try adding one new food to your repertoire each week. Children and mates may balk at first, but taking them shopping with you and letting them choose sometimes nips objections in the bud.

Using Churnas: Special Spicy Blends for Your Doshas · *Churnas* are special Ayurvedic combinations of spices blended with the individual doshas in mind. To use a churna, you simply sprinkle the mixture on your food at least once a day, just like salt and pepper. Churnas are the quick and easy way to season soups, stews, and vegetable dishes. Used generously, they turn any dish into instant curry. You can buy vata, pitta, and kapha churnas from the suppliers listed in our "Mail Order Suppliers" section. Or you can use the following formulas to make your own churnas. Buy powdered herbs individually at a health food store or Indian grocery, combine, and keep in a handy shaker jar.

- *Vata Churna:* Use this from late fall to late winter, depending on the severity of the climate you live in. Combine one teaspoon each powdered cinnamon, cumin, fennel, fenugreek, and ginger with ½ teaspoon each salt and pepper. Try this with a sauté of vata vegetables, such as beets, carrots, and sweet potatoes. Melt one teaspoon of ghee in a pan, add ½ teaspoon of the churna, and then ½ cup of each vegetable; you may also add two ounces of cubed tofu. Serve over steamed basmati rice.
- *Pitta Churna:* Use this churna from summer to late fall to stabilize pitta. Combine 1 teaspoon each powdered cinnamon, cardamom, licorice, poppy seed, turmeric, and sugar with ½ teaspoon nutmeg. This tastes particularly wonderful sprinkled on toast on which you have spread a little ghee.
- *Kapha Churna:* Use this combination from early spring to early summer to stabilize kapha. Combine 1 teaspoon each powdered cloves, dill, celery, ginger, cumin, tarragon, and pepper with ½ teaspoon powdered garlic. For a zesty salad dressing, add one teaspoon of this combination to ⅓ cup each grape-seed oil, balsamic vinegar and white vinegar; serve over a salad of raw cabbage, alfalfa sprouts, sunflower sprouts, and arugula.

Smell: Aromatherapy

How do smells affect you? Try to be aware of which aromas make you feel happy, content, secure . . . fallen leaves, apple pie, burning wood in a fireplace, the salt air by the seashore? Seek them out often and fill your life with them. Also try aromatherapy, the use of specific essential aromatic oils, a traditional Ayurvedic treatment for correcting imbalances in the doshas. This therapy works by penetrating into your memory and breaking the pattern of imbalance that lives there—quickly, effortlessly, and pleasurably. Choose essential oils based on your dosha:

- *Vata* is calmed by warm, sweet, sour smells such as basil, orange, rose, geranium, and clove. Vata tends to be fearful when out of balance, and aromatherapy cultivates positive vata emotions of joy and inventiveness.
- *Pitta* is balanced by sweet, cool aromas such as sandalwood, rose, mint, cinnamon, and jasmine. Pitta's irritability and anger are replaced with creativity and enthusiasm with aromatherapy.
- *Kapha* responds to pungent aromas such as juniper, eucalyptus, camphor, clove, and marjoram. These fragrances stimulate kapha out of its cynicism and apathy and toward extroversion, sociability, and energy.

Using Aromatherapy

- There are many beautiful diffusers available in stores and gift catalogs; these usually use candle power to heat water containing the oils.
- Place a few drops of the oils into a special ring made to be placed over a lightbulb; this disperses the fragrance as long as the bulb is on.
- Make a spray with the essential oils and water (add a few drops of lecithin to get the oil and water to mix).
- Sprinkle the oil in your bath, or add to a carrier oil to use in massage as explained in the chapter devoted to Step 5.

Precautions. Never take essential oils internally. Also, be sure to dilute essential oils with a carrier oil before applying to skin. The most commonly used carrier oil in Ayurveda is sesame, which is particularly suited to vata types and vata disorders; coconut is preferred for pitta; and flaxseed or almond oil for kapha. For body or massage oil, the usual ratio is ten drops essential oil per four ounces of carrier oil.

Sight: Color Therapy

Color is actually light. Your eye picks up the various lengths of light waves that bounce off an object's surface and sends them to the brain, which interprets them for you as "red," "blue" and so on. It is light, therefore, that actually feeds your brain, particularly the area of the brain known as the hypothalamus. The hypothalamus regulates and controls your adrenal, pituitary, and thymus gland and your entire endocrine system. We know that without proper exposure to light, disorders develop. The healthiest form of light is sunlight, or full-spectrum artificial light that mimics sunlight. Because many people spend most of their time indoors, they are starving for natural light. In addition to the light found in nature, humans also seem to crave the kinds of visual feasts that nature provides. To give your brain's visual center the nourishment it needs:

- Try to get outdoors for at least twenty minutes every day (even if it isn't a sunny day, you will still be exposed to natural light); take a short walk, sit in an outdoor café, play with your kids.
- Try to sit in a room with a window that lets in as much natural sunlight as possible into your home and workplace.
- Simply looking at natural scenes such as a stand of trees, ponds, streams, and other vegetation fosters positive feelings such as friend-liness and elation and discourages negative feelings such as sadness and fear. Adding more nature to your life—a walk by the river or in a park or garden, a living plant in your work space, a beautiful flower bouquet—could prove to be a potent stress reliever and beauty en-hancer.

Dosha-Specific Colors · Another beautifying tactic is to emphasize cer-tain specific colors in your surroundings (furnishings, wall and floor cov-erings, clothing, and so on) to help balance your doshas. The color messages sent by light waves affect the doshas, and hence your health, mood, and well-being:

- *Vatas* do best with pastel colors because they encourage calmness and serenity. Golden hues, yellow, orange, and white; small amounts of red, green, blue, and violet are also stabilizing and flattering. If you are vata, avoid black, gray, brown, and all dark colors.

- *Pittas* do best with white, green, and blue, which cool down their fiery intensity; gray and brown may be used in small amounts. Pittas should avoid strong, bright colors such as red and black and favor cooling silver rather than gold jewelry.
- *Kaphas* do best with rich warm colors such as red, orange, and golden yellows; purples usually complement their skin tones. Black, gray, and brown may be used in lesser amounts. Avoid white, pink, and pale green or blue.

Hearing: Sound Therapy

Sounds are vibrations—moving waves of molecules of air intercepted by your eardrums, transferred to three tiny bones in your ear, to fluid, to membranes, and finally to tiny hairs and auditory nerves that transmit the signal to the brain for interpretation. Thus, you "hear" with your ears and brain. But you also "feel" sound vibrations with all your body, which functions as a kind of reciprocal tuning fork, as you know if you have ever attended a live concert with a booming bass, or chanted "Om" solo or with a group.

Music is an organized form of sound and can directly affect mood, brain waves, and body chemistry. It has been found to enhance immune function, improve thinking ability; improve sleep, exercise, and work performance; help speed recovery from heart attacks and strokes; reduce side effects of chemotherapy; ease chronic pain; reduce the amount of anesthesia required during surgery; and reduce the amount of painkiller required during childbirth. If music is powerful enough to do all that, imagine what it could do for a few blemishes or wrinkles!

Raga (RAH-gah), the traditional form of Hindu music, means "musical color" in Sanskrit. With the upsurge of interest in Ayurveda, several companies have produced CDs and cassettes of ragas designed to balance the doshas. For example, Maharishi Ayur-Ved has produced a twenty-four-hour series of ragas that has been tested and shown to calm the nervous system and increase alpha brain waves associated with a relaxed, alert state of mind. They are based on the observation that different times of day have different vibratory qualities. The early morning, when the day is fresh and birds awaken and the dew is on the leaves, vibrates at a different frequency, for instance, than midday or the deep, dark velvet of late night. In this form of music, called Gandharva-Veda, ragas are based on these changing rhythms of the day that coincide with the doshas. In the following chapters, we recommend Gandharva-Veda to help solve common problems of the face, skin, hair, and weight control.

If you'd like to start working with sounds as part of your overall beauty and weight control program, try these tips:

- For a taste of how profoundly you can be affected by sound, wake up one morning to the sound of a screaming alarm clock. The next morning wake up to a recording of a babbling brook. Or compare the sound of a fingernail scraping across a blackboard to the purring of a contented kitten. One elicits a pounding heart or painful cringe; the other a gentle surge of joy.
- Experiment with various musical compositions to see how they affect you.
- Buy recordings of nature sounds to play when you are feeling out of sorts—agitated, blue, or angry.
- Buy a raga recording—if possible, a recording appropriate for your dominant or imbalanced dosha. These are available in Indian shops or large music stores with well-stocked foreign music sections and through the mail-order sources listed in the appendix. As mentioned above, Maharishi Ayur-ved sells recordings; Deepak Chopra's company also sells recordings of ragas composed for the three individual doshas.

Now that you've learned how to feed your body, your mind, your spirit, and all five senses, it's time to move on to Step 4, in which we focus more specifically on the face and complexion.

STEP 4

A Beautiful Face Every Day

*T*HERE'S NO GETTING AROUND IT: NO MATTER WHAT YOUR age, the skin on your face is often the most troublesome. And as time goes by, it betrays your age. Because your complexion requires more attention and tender loving care than the skin on your body, Step 4 of our beauty program is devoted to facial care, and in this chapter you learn how to make skin products and use them so you can then incorporate them into your Daily Regimen (Step 6). As you'll see, in Ayurveda it's quite easy and natural to achieve a clear, glowing complexion throughout your life.

Skin problems and needs vary according to the doshas. In this chapter, you'll learn how to make your own delightfully sensual and fragrant beauty products from fresh natural ingredients, and then how to use them in your Daily Skin Care Routine. For a more luxurious, elaborate facial that you can do monthly, see Step 7, "Once-a-Month Spa Program," which includes scrubs, medicated massage oils, and facial masks, again tailored to your particular type of skin. In this chapter, you'll also find suggestions for treating the most common complexion problems: excessively dry skin, wrinkles and lines, and very oily or blemished skin.

BASIC DAILY SKIN CARE ROUTINE

In this section you will find a daily routine for vata skin, for pitta skin, for kapha skin, and one for mature skin for all doshas. Before beginning a

❋ WHAT IS SKIN MADE OF? ❋

Your skin is the largest organ in your body. It is also quite complex. The *epidermis* is the outermost part and is made of layers of cells, the deepest layer of which, the basal cells, are always dividing. As they reproduce, the plump, fluid-filled cells push up toward the surface, replacing the dead, dried-out skin cells of the uppermost layer. The *dermis*, the middle part, contains collagen and elastin—protein fibers that inhabit the dermis like a mesh netting. This network of fibers is what supplies your skin with most of its strength and elasticity—the ability to withstand all the pulling and stretching it undergoes as we smile, frown, laugh, cry, and live under gravity's pull. Sweat and sebum together form your skin's "acid mantle." This thin film protects against bacteria and infection, retains moisture, and lubricates the skin surface. The deepest part of the skin, the *subcutaneous tissue*, is a network of fibers intertwined with deposits of fat. Your face and neck have very little or none of this type of tissue. Ayurveda works on all these layers of skin, from the inside out and the outside in.

skin care program, set aside time to know your dosha by taking the self-test in Step 1. Then choose your basic daily routine based on your predominant dosha. Your skin type usually coincides with your predominant dosha, but we have provided a checklist at the beginning of each routine to enable you to double-check and find the right facial regime for you.

The following Daily Skin Care Routines are designed to counteract the everyday effects of stress, environment, and time on your skin so that you can maintain what you have and relieve minor problems. Give these routines at least three to four weeks before judging their effectiveness, because skin needs 21 to 28 days to renew itself. The routines contain only two steps and require only two cosmetic formulas: a cleanser/exfoliant and a moisturizer/nourisher.

Commercial Ayurvedic skin care products are available (see "Mail Order Suppliers" section), but we feel that one of the most pleasurable aspects of Ayurvedic skin care is making your own cleansers, scrubs, and moisturizers. It's also fun to find special containers to store them in.

A word about the ingredients: You may notice that the ingredients called for in the recipes bear a striking resemblance to those recommended in Step 2, "Nourishing Your Body." That is because they are prescribed according to the way in which their taste and other attributes affect your doshas. The ingredients called for in the recipes are made of food and food products: herbs, flowers, and essential oils; vegetable oils, water, milk, cream, yogurt, and honey; powdered grains and nuts; fresh fruits and vegetables. Most of them are available in health food stores and Indian groceries; those not be available in your area may be ordered from the resources listed in the "Mail Order Suppliers" section of the appendix.

Remember, just because something is natural, it doesn't mean it's hypoallergenic, as anyone allergic to pollen can attest. If you tend toward allergies, do a sensitivity test before using any of the formulas recommended here. Make the skin care product, following the recipe, and apply a small amount to the inside of your elbow or forearm. Leave it on for twenty-four hours—if you do not see a reaction, you can safely use the formula. If you do notice a rash, you can test each ingredient separately (mix herbal powders with water to form a paste, and dilute essential oils with a base oil) and, once you've determined the culprit, eliminate it from the formula. For detailed information about the key ingredients, please turn to the glossary in the appendix.

Cleansing and Exfoliating

The road to healthy, radiant skin for all skin types begins with proper cleansing. Every day, you need to keep pores unclogged and remove makeup, dirt, pollutants, bacteria, sweat, and waste products that are eliminated through the skin. The catch is, you need to accomplish this without also removing your skin's natural oils and moisture (acid mantle).

In the Basic Daily Routines, we provide you with formulas for cleanser/exfoliants individualized to the three doshas. All are based on the following Master Formulas, which you vary as instructed for each dosha. We provide formulas for *Ubtans* (EWB-tans), herbal powders that are traditionally Ayurvedic. We also provide a simpler version, which we call a "Simple Cleanser"—to make it, all you need is chickpea flour and turmeric. This cleanser is tridoshic, meaning it is suitable for all skin types. This is the cleanser that Nancy and I use. We both have pitta skin and find that the soft powdery chickpea flour has just the right amount of abrasiveness for gentle daily exfoliation of dead cell buildup, and the turmeric is an anti-

---

❋ THE PROBLEM WITH COMMERCIAL CLEANSERS ❋

Most commercial soaps and cleansers are too harsh and drying, and they tip your acid mantle's balance from acid to alkaline. This is harmful to all skin types, but especially vata types who are already dry, and to pittas who tend to be sensitive. But even kapha types, whose oily skin spurs them to scrub away as much oil as possible to avoid breakouts, need to be careful. When you remove your natural lubricating and anti-bacteria layer, your skin reacts by producing more oil. Overcleansing also removes the acid mantle, your skin's natural shield against infection. Overgrowth of harmful bacteria is one of the main culprits in pimples and blackheads. As a result, overzealous cleansing can worsen the acne, rather than improve it.

---

bacterial to help unclog pores. This "Simple Cleanser" will leave your skin with a silky smooth softness, not dry or irritated, and impart a subtle golden glow. For those who prefer the feel of an oil-based product, we also provide formulas for a "Creamy Cleanser."

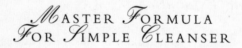

MASTER FORMULA
FOR SIMPLE CLEANSER

1 T. chickpea powder
1 tsp. turmeric

Combine ingredients and store in a small container such as a spice jar with a shaker top. To use, pour one teaspoon (or less) of this mixture into the palm of your hand or a small dish. Add enough liquid (the liquid depends on your dosha) to form a thin paste. With fingertips, massage all over your face and throat for one minute. Rinse with cool or lukewarm water.

MASTER FORMULA FOR HERBAL POWDER (UBTAN)

1 T. *chickpea powder*
½ tsp. *turmeric*
Various powdered herbs (amount and type vary according to your dosha)
Liquid (amount and type vary according to your dosha)

Combine ingredients and store in an opaque, airtight container. To use, pour one teaspoon (or less) in the palm of your hand or small dish. Add enough liquid to form a thin paste. Gently massage all over your face and throat with your fingertips for about one minute. Rinse off with cool or lukewarm water.

MASTER FORMULA FOR CREAMY CLEANSER

5 T. *base oil*
1 T. *each jojoba, avocado, sunflower, almond, and vitamin E oil*
4 T. *aloe vera gel*
1 T. *glycerin*
Essential oils (amount and type according to your dosha)

Place all ingredients in a blender and blend until creamy and fluffy. Store in an opaque airtight container. To use, massage a small amount all over your face and throat for about one minute; tissue off excess and rinse with cool or lukewarm water.

Moisturizing and Nourishing

The most important thing to understand about moisturizing is that the "moisture" refers to water. What we call "moisturizers" are in essence a mixture of water, which supplies the skin with moisture, and oil, which prevents the water from being drawn out of your skin by dry air, wind, and other elements. Moisturizers also minimize the appearance of wrinkles by holding moisture and plumping up the skin.

All skins need some form of moisturizer, even oily kapha types. Believe

THE PROBLEM WITH
❈ COMMERCIAL EXFOLIANTS AND PEELS ❈

Healthy glowing skin requires that the dead skin cells be removed, or exfoliated, daily. The Ayurvedic herbal powders and creamy cleansers provided in this chapter gently exfoliate as they cleanse, without stripping away natural moisture. They are preferable to commercial scrubbers, which contain synthetic chemicals and abrasive particles that can be too harsh for most skins, especially if used regularly.

Ayurveda also recommends against frequent use of commercial chemical "peels" such as retin-A, alphahydroxy acid, or glycolic acid. Although they are effective exfoliants, these products are too harsh and usually contain a synthetic form of these chemicals. They are particularly drying and irritating for vata and pitta skins if used every day. A better alternative is pure apple, lemon, or papaya juice mixed with water, but even they may prove too strong for delicate skin. The masks we provide in Step 7 are your safest bet.

it or not, rather than aggravating oily skin, using Ayurvedic moisturizer can help to quiet overactive oil glands. That's because they work differently than pore-clogging commercial moisturizers (see "The Problem with Commercial Moisturizers" page 76). The skin can absorb chemicals, and you want to be sure that what you feed it is pure and nourishing and has a beneficial effect on your doshas. The moisturizing/nourishing formulas included in this chapter are made of pure, natural ingredients selected for your skin type because of their ability to balance the doshas.

In the Basic Daily Routines, we also provide formulas for moisturizers individualized to the three doshas. All are based on the following Master Formulas, which you vary as instructed for each dosha. We provide formulas for a "Simple Moisturizer," which is simply a base oil plus essential oils and water. This is the moisturizer Nancy and I use every day. We only need a few drops, as long as we moisten the skin with water first, and massage the oils well into the damp skin. Nancy, who just turned fifty and sometimes suffers from dry skin in cold, dry weather, had been frustrated by creamy commercial moisturizers, even the high-priced brands with space-age anti-aging ingredients. No matter how much moisturizer she applied, on some days, her skin still felt dry. Since she switched to these

Ayurvedic formulas, made at the fraction of the cost of her store-bought products, she hasn't experienced one day of tight, dry skin.

We have included formulas for "Creamy Moisturizer" because you may prefer to use a heavier moisturizer at night, or if the simple moisturizer can not hydrate enough, especially if you have very dry skin or wrinkles, or if conditions in your environment are drying to your skin. Places such as New York City in the winter or dry desert-mountain cities such as Denver can really pull the moisture out of your skin. The creamy moisturizer contains cocoa butter and other pure ingredients such as aloe vera gel, which is known to soften skin.

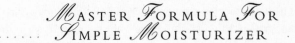

Master Formula For Simple Moisturizer

2 T. base oil
Essential oils (amount and type according to your dosha)

Combine oils and store in an opaque, airtight container with an eyedropper cap. To use, dampen face with tap water or bottled water and apply three to four drops of moisturizer to your skin. Massage gently until all the oil and the water is absorbed.

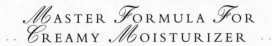

Master Formula For Creamy Moisturizer

6 T. base oil
2 T. cocoa butter
2 T. aloe vera gel
4 T. rose water
Essential oils (amount and type according to your dosha)

Place the oil and cocoa butter in a saucepan and heat until the cocoa butter liquifies. In a separate pan, heat the aloe vera gel and rose water. Place the contents of both pans in a blender and whip until creamy. Blend in the essential oils. Store in an airtight opaque container. Apply to your face and

THE PROBLEM WITH
❋ COMMERCIAL MOISTURIZERS ❋

Most commercial moisturizers contain substances that simply do not penetrate the skin down to the deeper layers, where you most need lubrication
and nourishment. They are usually just oil and water bound together with
chemicals called emulsifiers, which keep them from separating. They are
essentially a layer of grease that just sits on top of your skin, clogging pores
and attracting dirt. If the ingredients do penetrate, you get the synthetic
chemicals along with the moisturizing and nourishing effects. Be aware that
according to most skin experts, collagen complex in a jar has no effect on
the skin. Also be aware that commercial moisturizers often contain glycerin
or alcohol. These can backfire because glycerin pulls the skin's natural moisture up to the surface. Although this plumps up the outer layer, in the long
run it can cause dry skin if your deeper layers don't have plenty of moisture.
And alcohol is a drying agent, pure and simple. Check labels carefully if you
buy commercial moisturizers.

throat while your skin is still damp, and gently massage into your skin for
about one full minute.

Daily Skin Care Routine for Vata Types

Use this routine if you have vata-type skin or conditions (such as cold,
dry weather or a lot of stress) are creating a vata imbalance. You have vata-
type skin if your facial skin is:

- thin, with fine pores all over
- cool to the touch
- tends to feel slightly dry and tight, with some flaking in patches
- affected by cold, dry climate
- dark in color, or whitish or grayish-blue in tone

. . . and you sometimes experience the following skin problems:

- dull appearance, no "glow"
- roughness, chapping, cracked lips or feet
- dry rashes or dry eczema
- corns and calluses

Do the following routine twice a day, morning and night. If your skin is very dry, do not use any cleanser in the morning—just splash your face with plain cool or lukewarm water and pat gently dry. If you wear makeup, at night you may need to use a makeup remover first, such as sesame oil.

Cleanse

Simple Cleanser. Use the Master Formula (page 72), mixed with water or milk.
Herbal Powder (Ubtan). Start with the Master Formula (page 73) and add ¼ teaspoon each fennel, comfrey, lemon peel, tulsi; mix with milk, cream, or aloe vera juice.
Creamy Cleanser. Use the Master Formula (page 73) with sesame oil as the base oil; and three drops each of three of the following essential oils: rose, jasmine, geranium, cedar, sandalwood.

Moisturize

Simple Moisturizer. Use the Master Formula (page 75) with sesame oil as the base oil; add four drops each of geranium oil and neroli oil and two drops lemon oil.
Creamy Moisturizer. Use the Master Formula (page 75) with sesame, avocado, or walnut oil as the base oil; add three drops each of three of the following essential oils: clary sage, rose, cinnamon, clove, sandalwood, cypress, geranium, jasmine.

Daily Skin Care Routine for Pitta Types

Use this routine if you have pitta-type skin or conditions (such as hot weather, an excess of spicy food) are creating a pitta imbalance. You have pitta-type skin if your facial skin is:

- soft and glowing
- warm to the touch
- neither dry nor particularly oily, except for the T-zone (forehead, nose, chin), which is oilier and larger-pored than the rest of your face
- rosy- or peach-toned
- fair, with freckles

. . . and you sometimes experience the following skin problems:

- inflammation, itchiness, rashes
- T-zone is excessively oily, with blackheads, whiteheads, pimples
- acne rosacea
- premature wrinkles
- discolored spots and blotches

Follow this routine twice a day, morning and night, unless your skin is very sensitive; in that case, use the cleanser only in the evening and simply splash on plain water in the morning. If you wear makeup, at night you may need to use a makeup remover first, such as almond oil.

Cleanse

Simple Cleanser. Use the Master Formula (page 72). Mixed with water or rose water.
Herbal Powder (Ubtan). Start with the Master Formula (page 73) and add ¼ teaspoon each aloe vera powder, coriander, cumin, manjistha, and sandalwood; mix with milk, cream, or aloe vera juice.
Creamy Cleanser. Use the Master Formula (page 73) with coconut or almond oil as the base oil; add three drops each of three of the following essential oils: basil, rosemary, lemon.

Moisturize

Simple Moisturizer. Use the Master Formula (page 75) with almond or coconut oil as the base oil; add with 5 drops each of rose oil and sandalwood oil.
Creamy Moisturizer. Use the Master Formula (page 75) with almond, coconut, or sunflower oil as the base oil; add three drops each of three of the

following essential oils: chamomile, gardenia, geranium, honeysuckle, jasmine, mint, sandalwood.

Kapha Daily Skin Care Routine

Use this routine if you have kapha-type skin or conditions (such as cold, wet weather, an excess of heavy oily food) are creating a kapha imbalance. You have kapha-type skin if your facial skin is:

- thick and soft
- cool to the touch
- moist and somewhat oily
- relatively large-pored
- pale
- slow to show signs of aging

. . . and you sometimes experience the following skin problems:

- dull appearance
- congested, with noticeably enlarged pores
- oily and shiny
- many blackheads
- cystic acne

Follow this routine twice a day, morning and night, unless your skin is very oily and the weather is hot and humid; then cleanse and moisturize three times a day. If you wear makeup, at night you may need to use a makeup remover first, such as sunflower oil.

Cleanse

Simple Cleanser. Use the Master Formula (page 72), mixed with water or milk.

Herbal Powder (Ubtan). Start with the Master Formula (page 73) and add ¼ teaspoon each mustard powder, aloe vera powder, cumin, and lemon peel;

❀ LIKE SILK ❀

What a lovely idea—using a silk washcloth to cleanse your face. In Eastern cultures, women have traditionally pampered themselves by using silk cloths for their bath. Processed silk imparts a soft caress and is best for delicate vata and pitta skins, while raw silk helps exfoliate kapha skin. You can easily fashion your own facecloth by hemming together several layers of silk (to provide heft), and then use it to apply and gently and thoroughly help remove any of the cleansers or masks you'll find in this chapter. Your skin will feel like silk.

---

mix with plain yogurt or lemon juice diluted with an equal amount of water.

Creamy Cleanser. Use the Master Formula (page 73) with jojoba oil as the base oil; add one of the following combinations of essential oils: five drops each lemon and cypress, or three drops each bergamot, cypress and juniper.

Moisturize

Simple Moisturizer. Use the Master Formula (page 75) with safflower oil as the base oil; add three drops each of lavender, bergamot, and clary sage oil.

Creamy Moisturizer. Use the Master Formula (page 75) with jojoba, safflower, or canola oil as the base oil; add three drops of each of three of the following essential oils: cedar, cinnamon, eucalyptus, frankincense, and sage.

Daily Routine for Mature Skin

The following routine, formulated to keep skin young, supple, and glowing, is suitable for all three doshas and may be used by anyone who has reached her fifties.

Cleanse

Simple Cleanser. Use the Master Formula (page 72) mixed with water, milk, or wheat germ oil.

Herbal Powder (Ubtan). Start with the Master Formula (page 73) and add 1 tablespoon each aloe vera powder, ashwagandha, haritaki, neem, and rose petals; mix with equal parts of wheat germ oil and milk.

Creamy Cleanser. Use the Master Formula (page 73) with sesame or jojoba oil as the base; add 4 drops each of the following essential oils: lavender, frankincense, and neroli.

Moisturize

Creamy Moisturizer. Use the Master Formula (page 75) with rice bran oil or ghee (clarified butter, see page 32) as the base oil; add three drops each of the following essential oils: lavender, frankincense, and neroli.

TREATING COMMON COMPLEXION PROBLEMS

When you are bothered by specific skin conditions, the Daily Skin Care Routine may not be enough. You will need the following more specific, intensive cleansers, moisturizers, masks, and other special treatments. In this section you'll find specific remedies that work from the inside out as well as remedies that work from the outside in. These practices are explained in Steps 2 and 3 and presented in the At-Home Spa Programs in Steps 6, 7, and 8. At the end of this section, we discuss the factors that accelerate aging and give you tips on how to avoid them. Note: Remember, because you are using fresh natural ingredients and no chemical preservatives, these products will have a shorter shelf life than commercial products. Refrigeration will extend their life, but for best results, use immediately or within a few days of preparation, if you are using fresh fruits or vegetables.

Excessively Dry Skin

Although skin that is very dry or rough is associated with aging, your skin can feel dry, tight, and even itchy at any age. Still, there's no denying that as we get older, dehydrated, poorly lubricated skin lets wrinkles take hold and makes them look worse. This type of skin trouble is due to an imbalance in vata, the dry, windy dosha. Dry, flaky or scaly skin is a re-flection of your internal condition and indicates that you have a dry, nervous electrical system. Ayurveda offers both external and internal solutions.

From the Outside

1. Daily Cleanser. Use one of the following cleansers:
   - Liquid Cleanser. In the palm of your hand, combine one table-spoon heavy cream and a few drops of fresh lemon juice. Gently massage this moisturizing cleanser all over your face and neck with your fingertips. Rinse with lukewarm water.
   - Herbal Powder (Ubtan). Combine one tablespoon each of the following powdered herbs: ashwagandha, citrus peel powder, fen-ugreek, haritaki, lotus seed, rose petal, shatavari, and tulsi. Mix with enough heavy cream to form a paste and use as you would any Ubtan.

2. Daily Mask: To keep facial skin soft and smooth and prevent wrin-kles, use this simple mask after your cleanser every day.
   - Squeeze the juice out of five limes and combine well with eight ounces of honey; store in a glass bottle. After cleansing your skin, apply this solution to facial skin and neck and leave on for ten to fifteen minutes. Rinse with cold water and follow up with a mois-turizer.

3. Lubricate:
   - Sesame oil facial. All doshas with dry skin benefit from a daily sesame oil facial (see Step 7).
   - Brahmi Ghee—for pitta skin: Mix together one teaspoon brahmi (gotu kola) and one tablespoon ghee (clarified butter, page 32); this is traditionally massaged into to the dry areas three times a day.
   - Tomato-coconut mask—for vata and kapha skin: Use this dry skin treatment during the spring. Combine one tablespoon of fresh tomato juice with two tablespoons of coconut oil. Apply to your face and throat and let dry. Rinse with cold water.

From the Inside · Follow the Daily, Monthly, and Seasonal Spa Programs (Steps 6, 7, and 8) for vata to help balance your doshas internally. The Five-Senses Therapies (in Step 3) may also be helpful, particularly blue-green and yellow-orange color therapy, which is beneficial for dry skin. Every other day, take one of the following:

- Carrot-parsley juice. Combine the juice of two carrots with the juice of one bunch of parsley; this should yield about four to six ounces.
- Herbal elixir. Combine one tablespoon each triphala and yogaraj with two tablespoons shatavari; store in an airtight container. The dosage is ½ teaspoon every other day, in ½ cup warm water along with ¼ teaspoon of ghee (clarified butter, page 32).

Wrinkles and Lines

Wrinkles can be superficial or deep, have various causes, and therefore respond to different treatments. Superficial wrinkles are the fine lines that etch our faces as we age. They are caused primarily by sun damage or other dehumidifying conditions and vata-imbalancing conditions such as cold wind or dry air, excess coffee, sweets, spicy food, and a lack of love or purpose in life. Avoiding and dealing with these conditions is the best way to reduce and avoid many of these fine lines in the first place, as is taking good care of dry skin—a prelude to lines and wrinkles.

Deeper lines and creases are caused by habitual facial movements such as frowning, sleep position, sun damage and other dehydrating conditions, and the natural loss of subcutaneous fat and wear and tear on skin elasticity through aging, anxiety, or worry. Family predisposition and thin body types experience this earlier because they have less subcutaneous fat to begin with. Round, plump, full faces with oilier skin tend to look younger and stay looking younger than women with naturally thin faces and dry or normal skin.

From the Outside · Daily Mask: Use one of the following masks before you do your regular morning Basic Skin Care Routine.

honey mask—for vata skin. Combine equal amounts of fresh lemon juice and honey; apply to your face and neck and allow to dry before rinsing with cool water.

- Creamy mask—for pitta skin. Combine equal amounts of coconut milk and whipped cream. Apply to your face and neck and allow to dry before rinsing with cool water.
- Garlic-mustard oil mask—for kapha skin. Prepare this stimulating mask ahead of time by frying four cloves of freshly peeled garlic in ¼ cup pure mustard oil until garlic turns black. Remove the garlic from the oil and store the oil in a glass bottle. Let cool and apply to your face and neck and allow to penetrate for fifteen minutes.

From the Inside · Follow the Daily, Monthly, and Seasonal Spa Programs (Steps 6, 7, and 8) to help balance your doshas internally. Vatas are particularly at risk for fine wrinkles and pittas for deeper lines. The Five-Senses Therapies (Step 3) may also be helpful, particularly blue-green and yellow-orange color therapy, which is beneficial for dry vata skin; and green and blue, which balance pittas.

Very Oily or Blemished Skin (Acne)

Most people consider acne to be the bane of adolescence, but adults can suffer from the annoying embarrassment of breakouts, even if they went through their teens blemish free. The signs of acne—red, inflamed pimples, whiteheads, blackheads—occur when oil glands produce too much oil (sebum), or oil that contains ama, the toxic by-products of poorly digested food such as junk food. Bacteria on the skin interact with the sebum and cause abscesses to form—inflammation and plugging up of the hair follicles near the glands. Infection may set in, which can eventually cause scars. In Ayurveda, most chronic adult acne is considered to be a superficial sign of an underlying pitta imbalance.

If you have mild acne with only a few intermittent eruptions, Ayurvedic skin care can help prevent future breakouts and treat existing ones. A type of acne called acne rosacea, characterized by a red, sensitive rash on the nose and cheeks, is also due to a pitta imbalance. Sometimes a kapha imbalance can lead to a type of acne called cystic acne or acne vulgaris, which is characterized by very oily kin, large pus-filled pimples, and deep scars. These severe forms of acne are both best treated by a professional Ayurvedic practitioner.

From the Outside · Be sure to keep your skin clean, but over-enthusiastic scrubbing may actually worsen acne. Avoid squeezing pimples, since this can spread infection and injure delicate, inflamed tissues. Using the following skin care formulas will also keep breakouts to a minimum.

1. Daily Cleanser: Use the following Ubtan or Creamy Cleanser two or three times a day.
   - *Herbal Powder (Ubtan)*: Combine one tablespoon each amalaki, brahmi, manjistha, neem, fenugreek, lotus seed, and white sandalwood. Use as you would any Ubtan, adding plain yogurt or lemon juice diluted with an equal amount of water to form a paste.
   - *Creamy Cleanser:* Use the Master Formula with jojoba or sunflower oil as the base; add one of the following combinations of essential oils: six drops each lavender and tea tree oil, or six drops each bergamot and lemon oil. Use as you would any creamy cleanser.
2. Daily lime juice degreaser—for kapha types: Use this weekly treatment before your Basic Skin Care Routine. Combine one teaspoon lime juice, ½ teaspoon honey and few drops of milk. Apply to the skin before cleansing to lessen oiliness.
3. Summertime melon soother—for pitta types: Use this treatment to help control acne during the summer, when the hot weather aggravates your skin. After completing your Basic Skin Care Routine, simply rub the inner skin of a piece of watermelon rind on your skin at bedtime and leave the juicy residue on overnight.
4. Weekly egg white mask—for pitta or kapha skin types: Use this mask once a week before your Basic Skin Care Routine, until the oiliness is resolved. Combine the white of one egg and a half teaspoon of fresh lime juice. Apply to oily areas and leave on until it dries; then rinse with cool water.

From the Inside · Acne is usually a sign of a pitta imbalance, so follow the Daily, Monthly, and Seasonal routines for pitta (Steps 6, 7, and 8). Because flare-ups are often related to emotional upset, pay particular attention to stress-reducing practices including meditation, abdominal breathing, and yoga (in Step 3). You may also find taking one or more of the following remedies to be helpful:

- Herbal remedy: Take ½ teaspoon manjistha with pitta-balancing tea (page 40) three times a week to detoxify the blood.
- Aloe vera gel: Take one teaspoon aloe vera gel every morning.
- Drink warm water frequently throughout the day.

PREMATURE AGING

It happens to everyone at some point in her life. You look in the mirror one day and realize: "I'm getting wrinkles! I'm getting age spots! My eyelids are hanging down over my eyes! I'm turning into my mother!" How does this happen? Our genetic endowment (our prakruti) and the type of care we give our skin certainly count a great deal. But as we go about our daily lives, our skin is exposed to many other factors that can accelerate aging and thus have a huge effect on our appearance. So, take the following into consideration as you make choices about your daily habits:

- *Sunlight*. There's no question that sun is the major culprit in skin damage and aging. If you have any doubts, just compare your face and hands—areas that get the most exposure to the sun—with your buttocks and the skin under your breasts—areas that get the least exposure. So, the biggest and simplest step you can take toward younger-looking skin is to keep sun exposure to a minimum and wear protective clothing and sunscreen when you know you'll be sending a significant amount of time in the sun.
- *Stress and Thoughts*. Who hasn't known someone who aged perceptibly in a short time after a tragedy? But little, everyday stresses can have a cumulative effect as well. According to Ayurveda, what's going on in your mind is always reflected in your face. We now know that thoughts and feelings release certain chemicals or prevent them from being released, and this influences the rate of aging. Stress can cause lack of sleep and lead to a tired, sallow-looking complexion because

most of the cell renewal occurs during sleep; it can also lead to cigarette and alcohol consumption, which wreak their own special havoc (see below). For Ayurvedic stress-reduction techniques, see Step 3.

- *Weather.* Extremes of heat, cold, wind, and low humidity can have a drying effect, particularly on vata skin, and sudden changes cause broken capillaries to appear. No matter what your predominant dosha, try to avoid these conditions or protect your face with clothing and creams, and use a humidifier during times of low indoor humidity.
- *Sleeping Position.* The pressure on your face causes mechanical injury by compressing certain areas. Sleeping on your side with your face squashed by the pillow exaggerates the crease from nose to mouth, vertical creases on your forehead, and creases under your eyes. Sleeping on your back is the best position for your face.
- *Facial Expressions.* Those deep wrinkles you see in the mirror were likely formed by habitual facial expressions. You wouldn't want to stop smiling because smiling actually makes you feel happy. But frowning and squinting you can do without. Consciously try to reduce tension and wear adequate sunglasses to prevent frowning and squinting.
- *Skin Abuse.* Overly zealous rubbing, scrubbing, cleansing, applying and removing makeup all pull and stretch the skin and harm its fragile structures. With the gentle yet effective formulas provided below, you don't need to scrub to get clean.
- *Smoking and Alcohol.* Cigarettes and alcoholic beverages deplete the body of nutrients, slow skin renewal and repair, increase wrinkles, damage collagen, and give your skin a sallow appearance. Following the principles of Ayurveda will help you feel your best without resorting to these or any other health- and beauty-depleting drugs.
- *Frequent Weight Loss and Regain.* Also known as the yo-yo syndrome, this can stretch the skin, damage connective tissue, decrease elasticity, and lead to sags, bags, and more prominent wrinkles. The weight control program in Step 8 provides you with a plan that will slowly but permanently lead to your ideal weight.
- *Nutrition.* Your skin can get damaged from exposure to dirt, smog, sunlight and other pollutants, but certain nutrients seem to offer protection. Beta-carotene seems to be especially protective against sun damage, and vitamin C is essential in building new collagen, the pro-

tein that gives skin bounce. Vitamin E and selenium work together to protect against sunlight and pollution. Calcium is key, too, in preventing wrinkles, sags, and a gaunt look: calcium is needed to forestall osteoporosis, the bone thinning that can shrink your skull and result in loose skin. Fortunately, the Ayurvedic way of eating emphasizes foods that are rich in these and other nutrients your face and skin need to stay youthful and fresh.

Now that you know how to lavish loving yet simple care on your face, the next step is to apply similar principles to the skin on the rest of your body—all twenty-one square feet of it.

STEP 5

Beauty Secrets for Your Skin and Hair

*A*S IS THE CASE WITH FACIAL SKIN, THE SKIN ON YOUR BODY needs care to stay looking good throughout life. As part of our comprehensive beauty program, Step 5 reveals how Ayurveda's ancient secrets can help keep your body skin soft, smooth, radiant, and touchable, and your hair lustrous. Because your body skin accounts for many more square inches of surface area than does your face, Ayurvedic body care affords you a great opportunity to lubricate and nourish your body and spirit, and in this chapter, we acquaint you with the products you'll be using in Step 6, your Daily Spa Program.

We tell you how to gently yet thoroughly cleanse and keep your skin moisturized with natural alternatives to harsh soaps and chemical-laden body lotions tailored to your skin and body type. You'll learn how to give yourself a soothing oil massage and how to give your hands, feet, and even nasal passages the special attention they deserve. And you'll learn about therapeutic herbal baths and safe sunbathing. We also provide recipes for simple, effective conditioners and color enhancers for beautiful hair.

Because body skin and hair can become imbalanced, we then provide suggestions for treating the most common skin problems—skin rashes, excessively dry skin, skin bumps, and cellulite.

BASIC DAILY BODY CARE ROUTINE

As with your facial skin, the skin of your body usually exhibits the characteristics of your leading dosha. That's why we have provided different daily routines for each of the three types of skin. Take a moment to refer to Step 4 (page 69) and review the characteristics for each type of skin and the basics of cleansing and moisturizing. Then choose whatever routine is appropriate to your body's skin type. Before you cleanse and moisturize the body, you should first give youself an oil massage called Abhyanga.

Oil Massage (Abhyanga)

In India, it is traditional to massage oil into the body before cleansing. *Abhyanga* works on many levels to slow the aging process of the skin as well as your entire body. Applying oil to your skin lubricates, protects, detoxifies, and rejuvenates your skin and nervous system, while soothing your endocrine system. The oil helps loosen and liquefy ama so that the toxins can drain into the body's gastrointestinal tract for elimination. The stroking promotes relaxation and helps drain the lymphatic system, which carries nutrients to your cells and removes waste products. It is an excellent antidote for modern stresses, and I recommend it to all my patients to help them achieve the balance that is the foundation for spiritual development and inner beauty. In my practice, I have seen how Abhyanga alone relieves people of most of their daily stresses—and it is wonderfully lubricating for their skin.

Once you've regularly treated yourself to Abhyanga, you'll understand why it is considered to be the crown jewel of rejuvenation, prevention, and longevity. It's so addictive that even my busiest patients find a way to set aside the time for themselves. People of all three doshas benefit from oil massage, except if your kapha is aggravated; in this case you should use a dry massage, described below.

How to Do Self-Massage · Even my most frazzled patients set aside massage time in the morning just for themselves. It's even nicer if you can exchange massages with someone. Abhyanga can take as few as ten minutes,

---

❀ WHICH OIL TO USE? ❀

For your oil massage, be sure to get cold-pressed organic oil from a health food store. Never use mineral oil or any other oil that is not digestible (remember, your skin is a digestive organ).

- Vatas use: sesame oil
- Pittas use: coconut oil
- Kaphas use: sesame oil, but only if they are in balance.

---

or up to twenty minutes if you work slowly and take your time. If time is short, give yourself a mini-massage that involves just the ears, feet, and forehead.

To begin, warm the oil (use ⅛–¼ cup for the whole body, depending on your size and preference) to skin temperature or slightly warmer to make the massage more pleasant and to help the oil penetrate better. I use a small ceramic cup placed on an electric coffee warmer. You may also put the oil in a small dish or container and set that in a bowl of hot water until it reaches skin temperature. Be careful not to let the oil itself get too hot to avoid burning and scalding. Begin at the top of your body and work your way down, and do about twenty strokes on each part of your body as described below.

First, apply a thin coat all over your body to maximize the amount of time the oil comes into contact with your skin. (See above, "Which Oil to Use?" for information about massage oil.) Then massage your face, ears, and back of the ears, using short, vigorous strokes. It is traditional to apply oil to your scalp as well, but I have found this strips my hair of body. If you have little or no hair or wash your hair every day, this may not be a problem; alternatively, you can give your scalp an invigorating oil-free massage instead (see page 101). Proceed to your neck and shoulders, using your fingers and the palms of your hands. Then massage your upper arms and lower arms, using long back-and-forth strokes. Use a circular motion for your joints, including shoulders. Massage your chest and abdomen, using a clockwise motion. Next, massage your hip joints, buttocks, legs (again using long strokes), and then the ankles and soles of your feet.

✤ DRY MASSAGE (GARSHANA) ✤

If you are a kapha type or if your kapha is aggravated, give yourself an invigorating dry massage every day instead of an oil massage. Follow the directions for Abhyanga, above, using silk gloves designed for dry body rubs and sold at bath shops. Or you can easily make a simple mitt from a piece of silk that you have folded over and sewn to form a pocket. You may also use chickpea flour available at health food stores; rub this on your skin with the silk gloves or your bare hands.

If possible, leave the oil on your skin while you do some light exercise, such as yoga. Then, taking care to avoid slipping on the oil, wash it off in the bath or shower. You may use a mild soap, but I strongly recommend you use chickpea powder paste (see "Dry Massage (Garshana)," above). The paste will leave a slight protective film of the oil on your skin and exfoliate it so that it feels silky soft and smooth like your skin has never felt before. There is no need for additional moisturizer if you leave a thin film of oil on your body, which is what the chickpea powder does.

Cleansing

The next step in skin care is cleansing, which is a meaningful, joyous ritual in India. Indians traditionally sing or chant during the bath, in order to further purify and beautify the spirit and body. Depending on your lifestyle and on the weather, you should bathe or shower at least once a day (and by all means, sing or pray while you do so). As you'll see in the Daily Routines in Step 6, Ayurveda recommends that you bathe or shower in the morning, before meditation and after a calming self-massage with oil or a stimulating dry massage.

Master Formulas for Cleanser/Exfoliants

As is the case with facial skin, Ayurveda recommends that instead of soap, you use a paste made of finely ground flour and herbs. In this chapter, we provide formulas that are less intense versions of the same pastes recommended for facial skin care in Step 4. The Simple Cleanser is suitable for all three skin types. The Ubtans start out with the Simple Cleanser as a foundation, but you add a variety of powdered herbs according to your dosha.

· · · · · · *S*IMPLE *B*ODY *C*LEANSER · · · · ·

4 T. *chickpea flour*
1 tsp. *turmeric*
Liquid to form a paste (according to your dosha; use sesame oil if you have not performed the self-massage).

Combine ingredients and store in an opaque airtight container, preferably one that is unbreakable.

To Use the Cleansing Pastes · Stand or sit in a dry bathtub, (a bath seat makes this more comfortable). Take a small amount of the powder in your hand and add enough of the specified liquid to form a paste. Apply the paste to your body, beginning with one foot and working your way up to the ankle, calf, and thigh. Use a firm yet gentle circular motion to stimulate circulation and scrub those dead skin cells away. Keep massaging until the paste turns dry and starts to fall away. Take another portion of the paste and do the other leg. Then do buttocks, belly, hips, shoulders, neck and throat, arms, and face. If you are in a hurry, you may just concentrate on trouble spots—knees, back of upper arms, elbows, shoulders, thighs, and hips—and do a full body scrub once a week. These pastes are gentle enough to use on the genital area, but if you prefer, you may use a mild or moisturizing soap, such as olive oil soap, castile soap, or neem soap. Avoid deodorant soaps, which leave a filmy residue.

When you have finished scrubbing, shower the crumbs away, using comfortably warm water; follow with a cooler final rinse if you like—this will be more invigorating. Your skin will feel amazingly soft, smooth, and silky, with a pleasant tingle and a rosy glow, thanks to the boost in circulation. Pat yourself dry, and you are ready to apply moisturizing oil or lotion. This process is admittedly somewhat messy, and it may take you a while to get the coordination of it. But it will be worth it.

Moisturizing

In Ayurveda, you use pure and simple vegetable base oils combined with essential oils to keep your skin soft and supple. The formulas we recommend contain the same ingredients as the facial moisturizers in Step 4 but require proportionately less essential oils because those proportions would be too intense to use all over your body. One of the formulas is for a light body oil made of a base oil and a few drops of essential oils appropriate for your dosha; the other is for a thicker creamy body lotion that is more elaborate. Both are completely natural and easy to make.

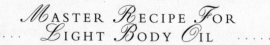

MASTER RECIPE FOR LIGHT BODY OIL

4 T. base oil
Essential oils (according to your dosha)

Combine ingredients and store in an opaque airtight container, preferably unbreakable.

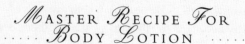

MASTER RECIPE FOR BODY LOTION

12 T. base oil
2 T. cocoa butter
2 T. aloe vera gel
4 T. rose water
Essential oils (according to your dosha)

Place the oil and cocoa butter in a saucepan and heat until the butter liquifies. In a separate pan, heat the aloe vera gel and rose water. Place the contents of both pans in a blender and whip until creamy. Add the essential oils. Store in an airtight opaque container.

To Use Body Oils and Lotions · For maximum effectiveness, apply the oil or lotion while your body is still damp from your bath or shower. You

may either want to skip towel drying and apply moisturiz
wet skin, or keep a spray bottle of water handy to redampen your skin. In
any case, use a small amount and massage in the moisturizer until it is well
absorbed.

Vata Daily Skin Care Routine

If your skin tends to be dry, follow this routine at least once a day.

Cleanse

Simple Body Cleanser. Combine the powder (page 93) with water or milk.
Herbal Powder (Ubtan). To the Simple Cleanser (page 93) add ¼ teaspoon
each aloe vera powder, fennel, coriander, comfrey, cumin, lemon peel,
licorice, manjistha, tulsi, and sandalwood; combine with milk, cream, or
aloe vera juice.

Moisturize

Light Body Oil. Use the Master Formula (page 94) with sesame oil as the
base; add four drops each of geranium oil and neroli oil and two drops
lemon oil.
Body Lotion. Use the Master Formula (page 94) with sesame, avocado, or
walnut oil as the base oil; add 3 drops each of three of the following essential
oils: clary sage, rose, cinnamon, clove, sandalwood, cypress, geranium, jasmine.

Pitta Daily Skin Care Routine

If your skin tends to be sensitive, follow this routine at least once a day.

Cleanse

Simple Body Cleanser. Combine the powder (page 93) with water or rose
water.
Herbal Powder (Ubtan). To the Simple Cleanser (page 93) add ¼ teaspoon
of each aloe vera powder, coriander, calamus, comfrey, cumin, elder flow-

ers, fenugreek, lemon peel, licorice, manjistha, nutmeg, tulsi, sandalwood, and vertiver; combine with water or pitta tea (see page 40).

Moisturize

Light Body Oil. Use the Master Formula (page 94) with almond or coconut oil as the base; add five drops each of rose oil and sandalwood oil.
Body Lotion. Use the Master Formula (page 94) with almond, coconut, or sunflower oil as the base oil; add three drops each of three of the following essential oils: chamomile, gardenia, geranium, honeysuckle, jasmine, mint, sandalwood.

Kapha Daily Skin Care Routine

If your skin tends to be oily, follow this routine at least once a day.

Cleanse

Simple Body Cleanser. Combine the powder (page 93) with water or milk. If you want your cleanser to be extra stimulating, add a few drops of mustard seed oil.
Herbal Powder (Ubtan). To the Simple Cleanser (page 93) add ¼ teaspoon each aloe vera powder, trikatu, calamus, comfrey, cumin, lemon peel, licorice, manjistha, nutmeg, tulsi, sandalwood; combine with plain yogurt or lemon juice diluted with an equal amount of water.

Moisturize

Light Body Oil. Use the Master Formula (page 94) with safflower oil as the base oil; add three drops each of lavender, bergamot, and clary sage oil.
Body Lotion. Use the Master Formula (page 94) with jojoba, safflower, or canola oil as the base oil; add three drops of each of three of the following essential oils: cedar, cinnamon, eucalyptus, frankincense, and sage.

THERAPEUTIC BATHS

If you love long, hot showers and baths, you're not alone. Sadly, they can be detrimental to your doshas and your skin. Vata types in particular need to watch out because if the skin becomes too water-logged during prolonged bathing, it actually loses water—moisture—and becomes dry. If you are predominantly pitta, the prolonged heat aggravates your dosha and may make you feel dizzy, weak, and even nauseated. And kapha types may become so relaxed as to be lethargic.

However, you needn't give them up completely; baths can be wonderfully therapeutic as well as cleansing, if you follow a few guidelines. Avoid really hot water and soaking for more than ten minutes—both can be too drying for most skin. Avoid bubble baths and bath gels that foam because they behave too much like soap, which destroys the protective mantle of your skin.

If you'd like to boost the therapeutic power of your bath, there are many natural ingredients you could add. To use herbs, place a handful of either dried or fresh herbs (perhaps from your garden or that you have purchased at a farmer's market or health food store) in a square of muslin or cheesecloth. Tie the ends together and suspend the packet in the flow of water as you fill the tub, then let the bag steep in the bathwater. You can then use the bag as a washcloth to fragrantly and gently cleanse and exfoliate your skin. Another way to use herbs is to add a strong tea known as a decoction to the bathwater (see "Making an Herbal Decoction," page 98). To use essential oils, simply add ten drops (total) of the recommended oils to the bathwater and inhale deeply as you bathe.

Vata · To relax and balance your dosha, use chamomile, elder, lime flowers, or sweet flag dried or fresh herbs or essential oils.

Pitta · To soothe and balance your dosha, use lavender and fennel dried or fresh herbs or essential oils.

Kapha · To stimulate and balance your dosha, use pine, juniper, mint, rosemary, angelica dried or fresh herbs or essential oils.

All Doshas

- To relax sore or tired muscles or joints: add four cups of epsom salts.
- To cleanse and soothe skin: add one cup of oatmeal.
- To moisturize and soften: add one cup of powdered milk or rose water.

❋ MAKING AN HERBAL DECOCTION ❋

Use one ounce of the herb and three cups of water. Break up the hard, woody parts of plants—stems, roots, and bark—into small pieces so that there is a greater surface area for the herb to be more readily released into the water; boil for about ten minutes until the water is reduced down to two cups. Next add the rest of the plant—leaves and flowers—and cover and steep for another ten minutes. Strain and cool the mixture before use.

Sunbathing

Through many cultures in history, the sun was a god, recognized and worshipped as the life-giver it is. As long ago and far away as ancient Egypt, Assyria, Babylonia, Greece, and Rome, people sunbathed to renew and restore themselves. In recent decades, however, we have recognized that too much sun can cause skin cancer and accelerate aging. Now that the ozone layer is compromised and less able to filter out harmful ultraviolet light, we need to be extra careful.

There's no question that excessive exposure to the sun damages the skin all over your body and increases your risk of skin cancer and melanoma. But should you avoid the sun completely? No—that would be unnatural. Many people find it pleasurable and relaxing to be in the sun. It helps regulate hormones and our internal clocks, and it is a source of vitamin D, which is needed for healthy bones and perhaps to prevent breast cancer. According to Ayurveda, sunbathing improves your circulation and encourages sweating, cleansing the body of toxins.

Vata and kapha types benefit in particular, because of the warming and nurturing qualities of sunlight; pittas need to be more careful because the heat of the sun can aggravate this fiery dosha. Light-skinned people of all doshas need to be cautious as well. Moderation is the key—one half hour a day to fifteen minutes twice a week, depending on your skin color. And of course always wear sunscreen and avoid the midday sun.

Moon Bathing

Bathing the skin in moonlight is another Ayurvedic tradition. It is said that the pale, cool light of the moon is cooling and calming to the doshas. Pittas in particular are said to benefit from a moonlight stroll or simply sitting near an open window during the full moon.

TAKING CARE OF YOUR HANDS AND FEET

The skin on your hands is the most abused skin on your body because you use them so much and subject them to sun, cold, wind, water, chemicals. It is often said that you can tell a person's age more from her hands than from her face. To protect your hands, wear gloves when gardening, washing up, and other tasks as well as during bad weather. Carry around a small container of body lotion or oil and use it after washing your hands or being in water. Take frequent work breaks if you use your hands—do wrist circles and hand stretches to ease the buildup of muscle tension. A regular yoga practice will also help keep hands lithe, limber, and strong.

Similarly, we abuse our feet terribly with high heels, narrow shoes, and high-impact aerobic exercise. Strong, flexible, healthy, pain-free feet are the foundation for good posture and a mobile, independent life as you age. Feet can also be quite beautiful and expressive. Nothing keeps feet healthier and happier than a regular yoga practice, going barefoot at home or while walking on soft grass or a sandy beach, and wearing comfortable, supportive footwear. A regular soaking in an aromatic footbath followed by a foot massage doesn't hurt, either, and is a good quick alternative to a full body bath and massage.

Nighttime Treatment for Hands

As a nighttime beauty treatment, apply a generous amount of Creamy Moisturizer (see recipe in Step 4, page 75), or combine one tablespoon sesame oil, one tablespoon plain yogurt, one egg yolk, and one teaspoon honey and apply to hands. Wear cotton gloves overnight to improve penetration and avoid soiling your sheets.

Treatment for Nails

In Ayurveda, the condition of your nails is an indication of the condition of your health in general. If you have problem nails, we advise you to address your whole body-mind. Horizontal indentations or split, weak nails indicate low agni, or digestive fire. Vertical ridges, bitten nails, and dry brittle nails are signs of a vata imbalance.

A good general beauty treatment for nails is to soak the fingertips in a small bowl of warm massage oil (page 91) suitable to your dosha. After a soothing soak of about ten minutes, remove your fingers from the oil and massage the oil well into your nails and cuticles.

Therapeutic Footbath

Use a quarter of a cup of decoction of fresh or dried herbs (page 98), or three drops of essential oils for the footbath. If you are prone to calluses, use a pumice stone to rub away dead skin daily, while skin is still soft from your shower, bath, or soak. Pay special attention to the heels of the feet, where skin can become particularly hard and even crack.

- To relax vata dosha: sandalwood
- To calm pitta dosha: lavender and fennel
- To invigorate kapha dosha: cool water and juniper, rosemary, and lavender

TAKING CARE OF YOUR SCALP AND HAIR

Hair is as important as your face, when it comes to physical beauty and the image you project to the world. Remember that your scalp is part of

---

❈ TAKING CARE OF YOUR NASAL PASSAGES ❈

No one sees the inside of your nose, so why should you care about your nasal passages? According to Ayurveda, clean, lubricated nasal passages are one key to health and beauty. Consider this: Modern allergists tell us we inhale two and a half *tablespoons* of solid particles every day! Think about it— each life-giving breath of air may also contain car exhaust, smog, formaldehyde fumes, pollens, and more. These unappetizing pollutants enter your nose, irritating the delicate nerve endings of your nasal passages; some of them even end up in your lungs.

Ayurveda offers *nasaya* (nah-SAH-yah-nah), a very simple technique that will lubricate and strengthen your cilia (the tiny hairs that line your respiratory tract and sweep away harmful particles), clean your sinuses, lubricate and protect the tender tissues responsible for your sense of smell, and improve your voice. To practice Nasaya, insert one or two drops of sesame oil into your nose, using either an eye dropper or the tip of your little finger; inhale strongly, so that the oil is carried into your nasal passages. We recommend that you do this once or twice a day; once you get in the habit, you'll wonder how you ever lived without it.

---

your skin and that the characteristics and problems you may have with your hair and scalp generally relate to your dominant dosha. So, vata types tend to have dry, itchy, flaky scalps with dry, coarse, frizzy, thin, fly-away hair; pitta types have sensitive scalps with soft, moderately thick hair, usually with reddish tones; kaphas have oily scalps (sometimes with oily flakes) and thick, oily, and shiny curly or wavy hair.

No matter what the style, length, or amount of hair, Ayurveda can help you have hair that is as soft, lustrous, and attractive as your prakruti allows. Like skin and fingernails, your hair is an outward reflection of the state of your inner health. Be aware that many factors affect your hair and scalp: bad hair days, weeks, and months can be due to age, general diet and health, season, climate, stress, anxiety. So eat a balanced diet appropriate to your dosha, reduce stress, and protect hair from too much sunlight and chlorine.

Massaging Your Scalp

Use your fingertips and thumbs to make small, firm circles all over your scalp. Then grab a small handful of hair and pull gently; repeat with another handful until your scalp feels relaxed and invigorated. If you like, you may repeat making the small circles all over your scalp. Or use a scalp massager with tiny projections to gently stimulate your scalp.

Shampoos

Did you know the word "shampoo" comes from the Hindu word *champo*, which means to massage? Unfortunately, as is the case with skin cleansers, most commercial shampoos strip away natural oils and tough up the outer layer (cuticle) of the hair shaft, no matter how "gentle" they claim to be. No wonder there's a proliferation of hair "conditioners" on the market. As you age, hair becomes more prone to dryness and dullness, particularly if you shampoo often.

We recommend olive oil shampoo, available in health food stores, for all hair types. You may want to tailor the shampoo to your dosha, by adding an herbal decoction (see "Making an Herbal Decoction," page 98). Prepare three cups of decoction; vatas use lavender or geranium; pittas use chamomile; and kaphas use rosemary. Add the decoction to ½ cup of the shampoo. This makes for a diluted solution that does not strip the hair of oil but which also does not create the satisfying sudsy foam with which you are familiar. Don't worry—your hair is still getting clean.

Conditioner

I have found the best conditioner for all types of hair to be half of a very ripe avocado. Rich in natural vegetable oil, avocado is a powerful remoisturizer and restores luster and manageability to dry, frizzy hair. You apply the avocado to your hair *before* you shampoo it. To prepare the conditioner, simply mash one-half of an over-ripened avocado with a fork, and add one tablespoon of warmed ghee if your hair is very dry. Dampen your hair and apply the avocado, massaging the scalp to the ends of your hair with your fingertips. Leave on for twenty minutes. Wash hair with a mild shampoo. For a final glossing, put a few drops of essential oil diluted with a carrier oil (the simple moisturizer or body oil works well) in the palm of your hand. Rub your palms together until the friction creates heat and warms the oil. Comb your fingers through your hair to distribute the oil through it. Your hair will be soft, shiny, and smell delicious.

Enhancing Your Hair Color

Is your hair looking drab and tired? Is there some gray that you're not happy about? Or are just a little bored and crave a bit of a change? You'll be glad to hear that you can use herbs as a safe, inexpensive alternative to harsh chemical colorants. Herbs are the perfect way to experiment because they temporarily revitalize and brighten your existing color without harming it, as ammonia or peroxide can do, and without risk to your health (hair dyes have been linked with increased risk of cancer). With the exception of henna, most herbs won't give you a dramatic effect—just a subtle highlighting and enriching. Your hair will look healthier, shinier, more vibrant. You may even tone down and blend in gray. Even this slight change can lift your spirits.

Herbal rinses work progressively—the change will occur gradually over time, so you have a great deal of control over the final effect. It also means you will need to apply them several times (up to fifteen or more at one session) until you achieve the results you want. The best way to do this is to re-use the mixture by leaning your head over a basin to catch the rinse as you pour it through your hair. Then, using a cup or pouring container, reapply the rinse from the basin. Remember: the results will gradually fade away unless you repeat the procedure regularly.

Before trying any herbal preparation, be sure to do a test run, especially if you have been using commercial dyes, rinses, perms, or straighteners because there may be chemical residues in your hair that will interact with the herbs. Either test the herbal preparation on the hair at the back of your head, where it won't be readily visible under most circumstances, or save some hair from your next haircut and use that as a test swatch.

- Chamomile brightener for blondes: use a chamomile rinse to brighten up drab blonde hair and to even out streaking from exposure to the sun. To make the rinse, boil half a cup of chamomile flowers in a quart of water for ten minutes; remove from heat and let steep a half an hour. Strain, and when cool, wash and towel dry your hair. Then pour the rinse through your locks fifteen times. Squeeze out the excess, place a plastic cap over your hair, and let the rinse sit for another fifteen minutes. Rinse with clear water.

- Rhubarb for golden tones: this works well for blonde and light brown hair. Simmer ¼ cup of chopped rhubarb root in three cups of water for twenty minutes. Strain, and when cool, wash and towel dry your hair. Pour the rhubarb rinse through your hair fifteen times and then rinse. This will give you warm honey highlights, which are heightened if you sit in the sun to dry your hair.

- Henna for warm red tones: henna is a time-tested herb that is no longer limited to the classic brassy-orange effect. Today there are henna-based products on the market that you might like to try; they range from deep dark red to warm delicate tones for blondes. Simply follow package directions. For a subtler effect, you might want to try this rinse: Add one tablespoon each of henna powder, chamomile blossoms, and vinegar to one quart of boiling water and steep for fifteen minutes. Strain, and when cool, shampoo and towel dry your hair. Wearing protective gloves, pour the rinse through fifteen times; for a more intense effect, leave on for fifteen minutes before rinsing with clear water.

- Sage darkener: To enrich and deepen dark brown or black hair, sage leaves are the preferred herb. You can also use sage to tone down and blend in gray. To make a rinse from sage leaves, add ½ cup of dried herb to one quart of boiling water. Steep for a half hour; let cool, and strain. Wash and towel dry your hair and pour the rinse through fifteen times or more. Squeeze out excess and let sit on your hair for another fifteen minutes. Then rinse with clear water.

TREATING COMMON SKIN AND HAIR PROBLEMS

Ayurveda says, "Know your skin, know your inner organs." The state of your skin, hair, and scalp reflects the state of your inner health, your doshas, and emotions. Your facial complexion is often the most expressive, but the skin on your body communicates, too. For example, hot, flushed skin indicates inner anger, and cold skin indicates fear or anxiety. Dry skin and dry, itchy, flaky-type rashes indicate a vata imbalance. Angry red inflamed rashes are due to pitta problems. Sluggish, oily, congested skin with moist blemishes suggest a kapha imbalance.

In the following section, you'll find Ayurvedic advice on common skin complains: skin bumps, excessively dry skin, and rashes. Please refer to Step 4 for suggestions about other conditions that affect both face and body.

Skin Bumps

Some women experience tiny bumps on their skin called keratosis pilaris, most often on the upper arms and buttocks. Kaphas are most prone to this condition. It is due to hair follicles becoming clogged with dead skin cells, and this accumulation feels like tiny hard bumps. The answer is to exfoliate the area every time you bathe or shower. You may use the chickpea and herbal pastes or the dry glove massage before your shower.

Excessively Dry Skin

Dry, itchy, flaky "alligator skin" is a common complaint during the winter (vata season). It is a reflection of your internal condition—a dry, nervous electrical system.

From the Outside · Use one of the following:

- Brahmi ghee: Mix together 1 teaspoon brahmi (gotu kola) and one tablespoon ghee (clarified butter, page 32); apply to the dry areas three times a day.
- Daily oil massage: Give yourself a daily full body massage with warm sesame oil. Sesame oil massage (Abyhanga, page 90) is a wonderful lubricant that softens your skin and works to correct the underlying vata imbalance as well.

From the Inside · Follow the Daily Lifestyle Regimen in Step 6 appropriate for balancing the vata dosha. In addition, take one or more of the following:

- Carrot juice: Combine the juice of two carrots with the juice of one bunch of parsley and drink four to six ounces three times a week.
- Herbal remedy: Combine one part each triphala and yogaraj with two parts shatavari (Asparagus racemosus); take ½ teaspoon every other day, in ½ cup warm water.
- Garlic milk. Mince one clove of garlic and add it to one cup of milk. Bring to a boil, and drink when it is cool enough. This restores the nervous system, is a natural sedative, and encourages the production of seratonin, a powerful neurotransmitter that regulates many functions in your nervous system.

Skin Rashes

Skin rashes in general are a classic pitta imbalance, a sign of a disturbed digestive fire, with redness, swelling, perhaps accompanied by fever and irritability. The rash may be infected and is worsened when exposed to heat and sun. Dermatitis and eczema are inflammatory skin conditions that indicate a severe pitta imbalance. When your digestive fire is low, ama forms, clogging the system and compromising your immunity. As a result, you become sensitive to substances in your environment such as detergent, jewelry, or cosmetics.

Other doshas can cause rashes too. Vata rashes are dry and flaky; this is a nervous disorder and is worsened by dry air and wind. Kapha rashes are wet and oozing and are worse in the damp and cold.

From the Outside · Use one or more of the following:

- Turmeric paste: The Ayurvedic remedy most commonly used to treat dermatitis and eczema is turmeric powder. Mix this herb with enough water to form a paste. Apply to the affected area three times a day. Leave it on until dry and then gently remove with a soft wet cloth. Use turmeric carefully, it will stain clothing.
- Papaya: Rubbing the inner skin of papaya over areas of the skin affected by eczema and dermatitis can bring some relief.

• Oils: Lubricate the skin with sesame oil (vata types), coconut oil (pittas), or any light oil (kaphas). Massaging the affected area with neem oil is helpful for all three doshas.

From the Inside • Following the appropriate Daily Lifestyle Regimen will eventually help correct the underlying dosha imbalance. Try to determine what triggers the rash, so that you can eliminate it from the environment. To avoid the rash becoming infected with bacteria or fungus, wash gently with mild soap (such as calendula soap) and water twice a day. Avoid strong soaps. Use soaps with perfumes or chemicals sparingly. Keep the affected areas away from water as much as possible. You may need to reduce bathing and washing and wear protective rubber gloves for hand washing of clothes or dishes.

In addition, you may find that a cool, damp cloth soothes the irritated skin; however, some rashes grow worse with cold application. Try not to scratch because it irritates already-inflamed skin. If you see signs of infection such as pus and worsening inflammation, see a physician. If the acute eczema returns again and again, it is probably a chronic condition and should be treated professionally. You may find the following natural remedy helpful:

• Pomegranate juice: Drink one cup of pomegranate juice, to which you have added one teaspoon of rock candy powder or organic sugar and five to ten drops of lime juice, two or three times per day.

This step completes the five preliminary steps of our program. Now that you have determined your doshas and become familiar with the Ayurvedic way of nourishing your body, mind, and spirit, and have your skin care products on hand, the next step is to put them all together into a Daily Spa Program.

STEP 6

Daily Spa Programs for Radiant Beauty

*I*N THIS CHAPTER, YOU'LL LEARN HOW TO BEST ORGANIZE YOUR day so that you reap the greatest good from the Ayurvedic practices you learned in Steps 1 through 5. Our Ayurvedic program not only provides you with the tools for creating health and beauty—it also provides you with a basic framework that makes every task easier because it is in synch with your body type and with the natural rhythms of the day.

In this chapter we explain the Ayurvedic belief that the timing of your activities—waking, eating, exercise, sleeping—is important to achieving and maintaining beauty. Then you'll find three daily schedules, one for each dosha, that show you how to integrate Ayurvedic practices into a daily plan that has grace, beauty, and practicality. Finally, we summarize Ayurveda's ten key steps to achieving inner and outer beauty.

The Daily Spa program is really about *sadhanas* (sad-HAH-naz) (see "Sadhanas" on page 110) and is your foundation for vibrant health and beauty. It paves the way to the following two chapters, where you will find more rigorous, deeper-acting programs to be done once a month and at the beginning of each season. These practices are simple, satisfying and effective. Listen to what this patient has to say: "Following the daily routine has transformed my life. I have more energy, more mental clarity, and my skin problems have gone away. Just doing the oil massage makes me feel more grounded now. I can move my joints better than I have before. It doesn't take very long, and I get so much out of it. Living my day this way is so simple and inexpensive; why didn't I do this years ago?"

❋ SADHANAS ❋

From the Sanskrit perspective, this chapter is about daily sadhanas. This is the Sanskrit term for the set of practices that are unique to each dosha. These are activities that keep you in tune with nature and thus keep your prakruti balanced. They are a part of your essential nature—much as fish swim, birds fly, streams flow, and wind blows. Daily sadhanas are your blueprint for living and for maintaining and achieving inner and outer beauty. Even the simplest task or sadhana can be enjoyable and reconnect us to the earth and all of nature.

PERSONALIZED DAILY LIFESTYLE ROUTINES

Everyone, regardless of his or her dominant dosha, follows the same general routine, but each dosha has its own particular timing for certain daily activities such as eating, exercising, and working. That's because in Ayurveda, *what* you do is important—but *when* you do it is important also.

Ayurveda explains this through the concept of daily dosha cycles: vata, pitta, and kapha are each at their peak during certain times of the day. Ayurveda divides the twenty-four-hour day into these time periods (they are approximate because they depend on the season and geographic location):

Vata times: 2 A.M.–6 A.M. *and* 2 P.M.–6 P.M.
Kapha times: 6 A.M.–10 A.M. *and* 6 P.M.–10 P.M.
Pitta times: 10 A.M.–2 P.M. *and* 10 P.M.–2 A.M.

For example, the morning is the kapha time of the day, when the body feels slow-moving, heavy, and calm. So everyone should be up by 6 A.M. or sunrise, because otherwise you find yourself too deeply in the kapha period and you will find it takes a lot of effort to get up and start the day. The middle of the day is more like pitta—it feels more active and energetic. During these hours you naturally work most efficiently. You are also best able to digest food, making it the best time to eat your biggest meal of the day. The early afternoon is the vata period. Studies have supported the

Ayurvedic observation that this is a time when most people think quickly and have the greatest manual dexterity—the characteristics of vata. Beginning at 10 o'clock at night, your pitta metabolism is doing most of its work. That's why we recommend that you get to sleep early so your body can devote itself to digesting everything you experienced during the day. Eating a substantial meal or engaging in intense mental or physical activity late at night means you are swimming against the tide of your natural cycles.

These daily sadhanas represent the *ideal* way of living. They are something to strive for, but few people can follow these guidelines perfectly every day. Real life keeps interfering! However, these sadhanas act synergistically, so we encourage you to incorporate as many as you can to get the greatest benefit. The more you can do, the easier it becomes to continue and to add to them. However, you'll probably want to begin by incorporating just a few of the practices into your current daily life, and then slowly add more. We know how difficult it can be to break out of established habits and replace them with new ones. But even small changes can have a profound effect, providing you with the motivation to make further changes.

Of course, many people have schedules and demands that simply prevent them from following these routines to the letter. Just do the best you can, as much as you can. Perhaps you'll just find time to meditate and do a bit of yoga in the morning and evening but will be able to follow the routine more completely on the weekend or while you are on vacation.

You will probably need to reconsider your priorities and get up earlier to give yourself enough time to accomplish your morning practices. You'll find that if you make time for these practices, you'll sleep better and use time more efficiently, be better prepared to face the day, have more energy, and be more productive. I often have to talk my patients into getting up regularly at 6 A.M. and going to bed earlier than they are used to. But once they do, they are true believers.

Vata-Balancing Guidelines

If you are predominantly vata, your most important goal is to maintain a regular daily schedule, and particularly to eat regular meals. This is difficult for the vata person to accomplish, but it is absolutely necessary if you want to have more reliable energy and sleep better. Once you start feeling and

---

CHRONOBIOLOGY AND THE
✸ RHYTHMS OF THE DAY ✸

It seems that we are genetically programmed to function best when we go with the flow of nature's natural rhythms. Chronobiology, the study of the natural peaks and valleys in the metabolic cycle, supports the ancient belief that eating, sleeping, and working are best accomplished at certain times of day and night. Chronobiology is discovering that hormones, enzymes, and neurotransmitters all ebb and flow at predictable times during a twenty-four-hour day. As a result, you are better able to process information, perform certain tasks, digest food, and so on, during certain times. Even drugs can have markedly different effects, depending on the time of day they are administered.

---

looking better, you may be tempted to slide back into your old irregular habits—resist!

- Vata types usually get the least amount of sleep, but you need the most in order to rest your frazzled, overworked nervous systems. You should get a solid seven to eight hours of sleep each night. You may sleep a bit later than the other doshas, but get to bed early and rise at the same time every morning—even on the weekends. In the morning, be sure to take time to do the oil massage and center yourself.
- During the day, be mindful of what you are doing—are you moving too much, doing too many things at one time, and thinking too much and too fast? Practice staying mentally focused and keep your movements steady and deliberate as well, particularly in the afternoon, when vatas tend to become scattered.
- You also need to avoid becoming overstimulated. Include periods of rest, relaxation, and reflection such as twenty minutes of meditation twice a day.
- Vata types don't do well in rainy, damp, or windy weather, so stay out of the cold and avoid these conditions whenever possible.
- Follow the food and spice guidelines in Step 2 to help you stay sta-

VATA: DAILY LIFESTYLE ROUTINE

	BASIC	OPTIONAL
Early morning	Arise by sunrise, without alarm clock. Drink warm water. Urinate and have bowel movement. Brush teeth and scrape tongue. Meditate. Do sesame oil massage. Do yoga Sun Salutation series at slow speed. Bathe/shower with warm water. Eat breakfast by 8 A.M.; a good vata-grounding meal would be cooked oat or wheat cereal with milk. Take short walk. Do calming exercises such as Tai chi or yoga, between 10 A.M.–12 P.M. or 4 P.M.–6 P.M.	Gargle with sesame oil. Lubricate nasal passages. Dry massage twice a week. Do additional yoga postures. Do breathing exercises.
Midmorning	Do active work; best time for meetings, communicating with others, doing chores and errands.	
Afternoon	Eat lunch between 12 P.M.–1 P.M.; cooked foods with a small fresh green salad and fresh fruits are best. Take short walk. Low-key work: thinking, contemplation, reflect on the day. Tea break at 4 P.M. Continue active work.	

	BASIC	OPTIONAL
Evening	Eat dinner between 6 P.M.– 7 P.M. Take short walk. Engage in light, relaxing activity. Meditate. Go to bed by 10 P.M.	Breathing exercises. Aromatherapy. Yoga.

bilized, especially during fall and winter, the vata time of year. Drink warm teas and fluids throughout the day, but avoid caffeine and alcohol.

Pitta-Balancing Guidelines

When pitta predominates in your prakruti, you need to tone down your intensity and plan your day so that you stay cool and calm. Instead of hanging onto your need to be highly organized, aim to loosen up and do some things out of pure enjoyment—forget about reaching a particular goal.

- When you are in balance, you have the most natural energy of all the doshas and can manage with six hours of sleep.
- Overexertion can burn out your fire, so allow time to relax and rejuvenate. You need to tone down your activities after 6 P.M.; meditating in the evening is especially useful for calming the pitta mind.
- Spending time among the cooling greens and blues of nature is especially beneficial for you. Plan to spend at least twenty minutes a day in a place where you are exposed to grass and trees or take a walk along a river, lake, ocean, or bay.
- Pitta types are unbalanced by hot/humid weather and conditions. You need to avoid overexposure to heat and direct sun.
- Because of your naturally high metabolism, eat whenever you are hungry, and don't skip meals or you will become cranky and irritable. Follow the guidelines in Step 2 for pitta-cooling foods and herbs, especially during the late spring and summer, the pitta time of year.

PITTA: DAILY LIFESTYLE ROUTINE

	BASIC	OPTIONAL
Early morning	Arise by sunrise without alarm clock. Drink warm water. Urinate and have bowel movement. Brush teeth and scrape tongue. Meditate. Do coconut oil massage. Do yoga Sun Salutation series. Eat breakfast by 8 A.M.; a light breakfast of grains such as rice or wheat with ghee, and fruit is best. Take short walk. Do exercise that is competitive and/or involves other people, before 10 A.M., or after 2 P.M.	Gargle with sesame oil. Lubricate nasal passages. Dry massage 3 times a week. Additional yoga postures. Breathing exercises.
Midmorning	Do active work; best time for communicating with others, creative activities, nonstressful work in late morning.	
Afternoon	Eat lunch between 12 P.M.– 2 P.M.; a good lunch would be a salad with raw fennel and a sandwich with almond butter. Take short walk. Do detailed work, communications, meetings, present creative ideas, make proposals. Tea break and snack at 3 P.M. Assess your performance and effectiveness, plan tomorrow's schedule.	

	BASIC	OPTIONAL
Evening	Eat dinner between 6 P.M.–7 P.M. Take short walk. Engage in light, relaxing activity. Meditate. Go to bed by 10:30 P.M.–11:00 P.M.	Breathing exercises. Aromatherapy. Yoga.

Avoid stimulating foods and herbs and, especially, artificial stimulants and drugs.

Kapha-Balancing Guidelines

Kapha types tend to be procrastinators—lethargic and slow to get moving. So the most important thing for you to aim for is a strict, structured schedule. On the other hand, you also easily get stuck in a rut, so you need to keep changing your routine slightly from day to day.

· Kapha types usually get the most sleep but require the least. Six or seven hours a night is plenty for you; excess sleep increases kapha, which increases inertia, which fosters sleeping, which increases kapha, and so on in a never-ending cycle. To break or avoid this cycle, "early to bed and early to rise" should be your mantra. Because you already tend to be sluggish, getting up after dawn (when the kapha part of the day is in full swing) makes it even harder for you to get going in the morning. You need to rise the earliest of all three types, and you must avoid staying in bed after 6 A.M. at all costs.

· Plan your day to include *at least* twenty minutes of vigorous physical activity. Every kapha benefits from early morning exercise to jump-start the system. But if you tend to put on weight, a common kapha characteristic, you absolutely require physical activity to stay trim.

· Kaphas feel heavier and sluggish in cold, damp weather, so do your best to keep warm and dry by avoiding these conditions.

· Pay attention to the food and spice guidelines outlined in Step 2 so you stay balanced, particularly during late winter and early spring,

KAPHA: DAILY LIFESTYLE ROUTINE

	BASIC	OPTIONAL
Early morning	Arise by sunrise without alarm clock, preferably earlier. Drink warm water. Urinate and have bowel movement. Brush teeth and scrape tongue. Meditate. Dry massage. Do yoga Sun Salutation series, at top speed. Bathe/shower with warm water. Eat light breakfast by 8 A.M., such as fruit and tea. Take short, fast walk.	Lubricate nasal passages. Additional yoga postures, breathing exercises.
Midmorning	This is the best time for you to do activities that are mentally stimulating and challenging.	
Afternoon	Eat lunch between 12 P.M.– 2 P.M. Take short walk. Resume work activities, especially those involving light physical effort. Tea break. Continue active work.	
Evening	Eat dinner between 6 P.M.– 7 P.M. Do strenuous exercise, such as walking uphill. Engage in consistent stimulating activity outside the home, with wind-down time. Meditate. Go to bed by 9:30 P.M.–10 P.M.	Breathing exercises. Aromatherapy. Yoga.

the kapha season. Eat a very light breakfast, if any, and a light supper, and drink warming teas and fluids during the day.

10 KEY STEPS TO INNER AND OUTER RADIANCE

In summary, here are the ten most important basic principles and practices to keep in mind as you go about your day.

1. Get the right amount of sleep. Sleep is one of the greatest health and beauty tools at your disposal. A good night's sleep and enough of it is crucial in rejuvenating the mind and body and in restoring a fresh appearance. In Ayurveda, proper sleep is paramount because it helps you mentally and physically digest everything you took in that day. In general, you should be up before the sun rises and asleep by 10 P.M. in order to take advantage of your body's natural rhythms and functions. If you have problems falling asleep or staying asleep, Ayurveda offers several techniques that relieve insomnia (see "Treating Insomnia," page 120). Instead of "knocking you out," as habit-forming conventional medicines tend to do, Ayurvedic practices and remedies encourage the body to drift into a natural, restful sleep.

2. Pay attention to elimination. An Indian proverb says, "One who evacuates his bowels in less than a minute and does not owe any money is the happiest person." In Ayurveda, it is important to have at least one bowel movement every day, preferably in the morning before meditation. One of the worst things you can do for health and beauty is to ignore the urge when you have to go to the bathroom. Eliminating waste products reduces the accumulation of ama, the toxic gunk that clogs your system and dulls your inner glow and slows down your metabolism. One of the wonderful things about Ayurveda is that its practices bring about regularity, without the need for the strong laxative jolt of coffee in the morning.

3. Avoid suppressing any other natural biological urges, including sneezes, thirst, hunger, coughs, yawns, tears, laughter, runny nose,

flatus, and urine. Ayurveda believes suppression can lead to diseases and poor appearance later on.

4. Get out in the fresh air and sunlight every day for at least twenty minutes. Take a walk or sit outdoors when you eat lunch. Being around nature is a traditional Ayurveda prescription, and recent studies support the observation that nature is good for your health. Never shape your day so that you are constantly indoors or in your car.

5. Sip water throughout the day. Ayurveda believes that it is best to drink pure spring water or filtered water that has been boiled for ten minutes. After boiling, let the water cool to room temperature and sip one or two ounces every half hour to restore balance to your bioenergetic body (a total of two to four cups of boiled water per day). This practice of drinking bioenergetically treated water is inexpensive, easy, and very powerful for balancing all three doshas. The boiling is not for the purpose of purifying the water; it is an energetic treatment. Boiling creates movement which stimulates vata; it creates heat, which stimulates pitta; and it creates steam, which stimulates kapha.

6. Clean your tongue in the morning, not just your teeth. After brushing your teeth, scrape the morning residue of ama from your tongue every day. It is traditionally recommended that vatas use a gold tongue scraper, pitta use silver, and kapha use copper (for suppliers, see "Mail Order Suppliers"). Any body type can use a stainless steel scraper; plastic tongue scrapers are also available at pharmacies. Alternatively, you can simply use your toothbrush, making forward-moving strokes beginning at the back of the tongue. Avoid scraping too far back on your tongue to prevent triggering the gag reflex, an unpleasant way to start the day. Scraping not only stimulates your digestive fire; it also removes bacteria from your tongue.

7. Use television prudently, if at all. Television can have a negative or a positive effect, depending how you use it. For example, there are many healing and educational videotapes available on a variety of subjects from yoga to visualization to laughter. But if you watch too much, it can overstimulate your sight and hearing, which increases vata; because it is a passive activity, it increases kapha.

8. Ayurveda believes that sex is a wonderful part of life and can enhance spirituality. Generally, it is thought that having sexual relations twice a week is healthy, but you should simply obey whatever natural urges you have, provided you are in a balanced state.

9. Love, joy, kindness, honesty, compassion, generosity, understanding, courage, and clarity in our relationships and everyday life are important to good health, long life, and inner radiance. But there is more to life than these positive emotions, and when your doshas are balanced, you are able to feel and express sadness, anger, or hurt while your inner beauty still shines through.

10. Ayurveda is built on a diet and lifestyle in relation to your environment. You need to create a daily routine that takes care of your needs first and foremost, but with awareness and reverence for the environment and the fragility of our planet. In Sanskrit, the word *dharma* (DAR-mah) refers to the unwritten code of conduct that makes us aware of the difference between right and wrong. If you violate this code, your life and anything you accomplish or possess will be devoid of beauty, grace, and happiness. But if you adhere to this code, you will enjoy a life of abundance and beauty, which is a reflection of you.

Once you have followed this Daily Spa Program for at least one month, you are ready to progress to the next level of our beauty program. In the following chapter, Step 7, we show you how to pamper yourself once a month from head to toe, inside and out.

❋ TREATING INSOMNIA ❋

If you need an alarm clock to wake up every morning; if you don't wake up refreshed and energetic; if you sleep fitfully and wake up tired, Ayurvedic self-care measures and remedies can help you restore a normal sleep schedule and awaken refreshed rather than exhausted. Because insomnia is characteristic of a vata imbalance, following a vata-stabilizing Daily Spa Program will restore balance and go a long way toward restoring your ability to get a good night's sleep. In addition:

- Establish healthy sleep habits: Adhere to a regular sleep pattern; follow a regular exercise routine; eat a light supper, and finish eating no later than 8 P.M.; avoid caffeine (in coffee, black tea, sodas, chocolate, and some conventional drugs) for several hours before bedtime; avoid drinking alcoholic beverages in the evening; avoid stimulating nighttime activities; create a bedtime ritual that cues your body for sleep and disengages the mind from daytime problems and thoughts; use ear plugs if your bedroom is noisy; make sure your bedroom is dark; and keep your bedroom for two things only—sleep and sex.
- Do yoga. Gentle yoga stretches before going to bed are a good way to dissipate the tensions of the day. Meditation and breathing and relaxation exercises also calm the body-mind.
- Sleep with your head toward the east for relaxing, meditative sleep, and toward the south for recharging and healing. If your head faces the west, you may suffer from a restless type of sleep, and if your head faces north, it is said to drain you of energy.
- Use aromatherapy. Sweet, warm aromas, such as basil, orange, rose, geranium, and cloves work wonders when inhaled just before bedtime and during sleep.
- Use music therapy: Listen to the late afternoon Gandharva-vedic raga from 4 to 7 P.M., and the sunset raga from 7 P.M. to 10 P.M.; if you are still awake, listen to the late-night raga.
- Apply Brahmi oil (gotu kola herb in a coconut oil base, available from suppliers listed in the appendix) to your forehead, soles of the feet, and navel area before retiring.
- Try one of these herbal remedies:
  - ★ Mix 1 teaspoon ashwaghanha (Withania somnifera) and 1 pinch each cardamom and saffron with 1 cup hot milk.
  - ★ Mix 1 teaspoon ashwagandha and ¼ teaspoon each jatamansi (valerian) and brahmi (gotu kola) with 1 cup warm milk.
  - ★ Mix ½ teaspoon each cardamom and ghee and ⅛ teaspoon nutmeg with one cup warm milk.
  - ★ Sauté ⅛ teaspoon nutmeg and ½ teaspoon jaggery (brown sugar) in one teaspoon ghee (clarified butter, see page 32); combine with one cup heated milk.

Precautions: Chronic insomnia due to physical illness or emotional imbalance requires professional evaluation and counseling. Seek medical care if you experience insomnia for more than seven consecutive days or if you have a painful medical condition that is keeping you from getting a good night's rest.

STEP 7

Once-a-Month Spa Program

FOLLOWING THE DAILY SPA PROGRAM IN STEP 6 WILL MAKE a big difference in the way you look and feel. But it can only do so much. That's why we recommend that once a month you do a more thorough external and internal cleansing, purification, and rejuvenation. The treatments in this chapter will renew your energy, lift your spirits, and pamper your skin and body from head to toe, inside and out.

This step consists of two parts. The first part is a two-day external program that deep cleans and rejuvenates your face and skin; it requires just an hour or two each day. These treatments will make you feel quite pampered and are easy to do. The second part is a six-day program of *panchakarma* (PAHN-cha-KAR-mah)—internal treatments that cleanse and purify your whole system. These treatments can be quite powerful, so this part of the program is not for everyone. **Do not attempt the internal cleansing program unless you have followed the Daily Spa Routine for at least one month**.

EXTERNAL SPA PROGRAM: FACE AND SKIN

To keep your skin in the best condition, all skin types need something extra beyond the daily complexion and skin care routines outlined in Steps 4 and 5. These monthly routines add several procedures to those programs.

In addition to cleansing and moisturizing, you also give yourself a facial massage and full-body massage; treat your face to an herbal steam; exfoliate your entire body with an invigorating scrub; and apply a deep cleaning, nourishing, calming, cooling, or invigorating mask. There are three routines—one for each dosha. If you have mature skin, you may notice that it has become drier as you have gotten older; if so, follow the procedure for either vata skin or mature skin.

We have divided the two days so that you do your face on one day, your body on the next. You'll get wonderful results for your skin and find it wonderfully nurturing for your spirit as well. This external program is more effective and rewarding if you try to follow an easy, relaxed schedule. Eat pure, simple foods such as vegetables, rice, and lentils; try to meditate twice a day; do breathing exercises; and do yoga or other low-key exercise.

DAY ONE: PAMPER YOUR FACE

Today's spa treatment consists of these components:

1. Facial Massage with Aromatic Oil
2. Steam with Fragrant Herbs and Oils
3. Herbal Scrub
4. Fresh Fruit and Vegetable Mask
5. Moisturizer

1. Facial Massage with Aromatic Oil

Why is facial massage important? For one thing, the epidermis, or outer layer of skin, has no blood vessels. It depends on the fluid between the cells in the dermis to get its nourishment and to remove toxins and waste products. Facial massage helps increase the circulation to your dermis; this in turn benefits your epidermis and gives you a healthier, more vital, and glowing complexion. In addition, there are many sensitive reflex points (marma points) on the face and scalp, so this massage can activate the deep centers of your brain, soothe your entire body, and relax any unnecessary tension in the muscles of your face, neck, and shoulders.

Try this facial massage yourself, or trade with a friend. It's wonderfully luxurious to have a professional facial once a month, which includes a mas-

USING THE RIGHT MASSAGE OIL
❋ FOR YOUR DOSHA ❋

- *Vata Skin*: Use a base oil of 8 tablespoons sesame or almond oil, with 16 drops each of geranium oil and neroli oil and 8 drops lemon oil.
- *Pitta Skin*: Use a base oil of 8 tablespoons almond or coconut oil, with 20 drops each of rose oil and sandalwood oil.
- *Kapha Skin*: Use a base oil of 8 tablespoons safflower oil, with 12 drops each of lavender, bergamot, and clary sage oil.
- *Very Oily or Blemished Skin*: Use a base oil of 8 tablespoons jojoba oil, with 20 drops each of either lavender and tea tree oil, or bergamot and lemon oil.
- *Mature Skin*: Use a base oil of 5 tablespoons jojoba oil, 4 tablespoons calendula oil, and 1 tablespoon wheat germ oil; add 12 drops each of essential oil of lavender, frankincense, neroli.

sage of the face, neck, and shoulders. Select the appropriate massage oil based on your constitution, and if you like, you may add essential oils, also tailored to your constitution, for additional benefits (see "Using the Right Massage Oil for Your Dosha," above). First massage your body as usual; then concentrate on your face.

Doing the Facial Massage · Before you begin, tie your hair back or wrap it in a towel to keep it out of the way. Place some massage oil in the palms of your hands and rub your hands together to warm the oil.

1. To begin, place your full palms over your face for a few moments. Then draw your hands up over your face with soft, light strokes. With your fingertips, make sweeping movements up your neck and over your chin and jaw.
2. Making small circles with your fingertips, massage along your jaw, up your outer cheeks, and up to your temples. Stroke from the center of your face along the cheeks and up to the hairline in front of your ears.
3. Next, massage from the center of your forehead out to the temples,

then down the sides of your face. Press your thumbs or the heels of your hands firmly under the lower edges of your cheekbones.

4. Press your fingertips around your hairline in front of your ears; then move up around and to the back of your ears, pressing the points where your ear joins your skull. Squeeze your earlobes between your thumbs and forefingers, then work your way up and around the edge of your ear, squeezing with as much pressure as feels good to you.

5. Also press the following marma points: the point in the indentation between your lower lip and chin; the point where your eyebrows begin at the bridge of your nose; the "third eye" point on your forehead just above your eyebrows.

6. To finish, gently place the palms of both hands over your face, covering your eyes, and let them rest there for a few quiet moments while you enjoy the effects of the massage. When you are ready, let both palms fall away slowly, and rest as long as you like before going on to the next step—the herbal steam.

2. Steam with Fragrant Herbs and Oils

Steam cleaning is an ancient technique for purifying the complexion. It's quite easy to create your own at-home minisauna for your face. You may use plain steam, and this alone will help open pores, loosen blackheads, draw out pimples, and remove stubborn dirt and toxins. But in Ayurveda, it is customary to add fragrant herbs or essential oils appropriate to your doshas to obtain added benefits for your skin, body, and mind (see "Using the Right Herbs and Essential Oils," page 127). The fragrance boosts circulation to your face and helps coax out deep-down impurities such as dirt, toxins, and waste products, bringing them to the surface, where they can be easily removed. Fragrant herbs also lift your spirits, ease tensions, and balance your doshas, improving the appearance of your skin from the inside and the outside.

Giving Yourself an Herbal Steam · Heat one quart of water in a saucepan. If you are using herbs add one cup of the herbal combination that suits your dosha when the water has begun to boil. Cover, and remove from heat, and allow to steep for two minutes. If you are using essential oils, add

---

USING THE RIGHT HERBS
❈ AND ESSENTIAL OILS FOR YOUR DOSHA ❈

- *Vata Skin:*
  Herbs: licorice, chamomile, comfrey, rose, sandalwood, orange peel.
  Essential Oils: rose, neroli, chamomile.
- *Pitta Skin:*
  Herbs: licorice, sandalwood, chamomile, clover, comfrey, fennel, lavender, rose.
  Essential Oils: lavender, geranium, sandalwood.
- *Kapha Skin:*
  Herbs: fennel, lavender, lemon balm or lemon grass, lemon peel, lemon verbena, rosemary, sandalwood, dashmoola.
  Essential Oils: juniper, bergamot, cypress.
- *Mature Skin (all doshas):*
  Herbs: orange peel, fennel, ginger, mint, haritiki.
  Essential Oils: rose, neroli, chamomile.
- *Very Oily or Blemished Skin (all doshas):*
  Herbs: licorice, black currant leaf, burdock root, dandelion root, manjistha, yarrow.
  Essential Oils: rose, lemon, bergamot, lavender.

---

10 drops of the essential oil combination of your choice. Place the covered pot on a table over which you can comfortably lean (protect the table surface with a trivet). Lean over the pot so that your face enters the stream of vaporized water, and make a tent with a bath towel to keep the steam from escaping. Be careful you don't put your face too close to the hot water—this could cause scalding and lead to broken blood vessels. Steam your face for five to ten minutes. Pat dry, and you are now ready for your herbal scrub.

3. Herbal Scrub

Scrubs are used to remove dead cells (exfoliate) your skin, stimulate circulation, cleanse pores, and prevent blackheads. Used regularly, they impart a healthy glow and help stimulate healthy new cell growth. The Ubtans

✤ USING THE RIGHT SCRUB FOR YOUR DOSHA ✤

- *Vata Skin*
  Powder: Blend one tablespoon each of chickpea flour, wheat germ, almond powder, ashwagandha, haritaki, fenugreek, tulsi.
  Liquid: Use milk (powdered milk and water is acceptable), cream, or aloe vera juice.
- *Pitta Skin*
  Powder: Blend 1 tablespoon each of chickpea flour, tulsi, sandalwood, and rose petals.
  Liquid: Use milk (powdered milk and water is acceptable), comfrey tea, or pure water.
- *Kapha Skin*
  Powder: Blend 1 tablespoon each of chickpea flour, rice bran, amalaki, coriander, neem, sandalwood, and lavender.
  Liquid: Lemon juice diluted half with water or aloe vera juice.
- *Mature Skin (all doshas)*
  Powder: Blend 1 tablespoon each of rice flour, haritaki, ashwagandha, tulsi, licorice, orange blossom.
  Liquid: Use milk (powdered milk and water is acceptable), and honey or aloe vera juice.
- *Very Oily or Blemished Skin (all doshas)*
  Powder: Blend 1 tablespoon each of oat flour, ashwagandha, coriander, cumin, haritaki, ginger, neem, turmeric, and lavender.
  Liquid: Use plain yogurt.

and cleansers specified in the Daily Skin Care Routines are mild exfoliants. You may use those as part of your monthly routine or the more intense scrub formulas provided here. Unlike commercial scrubs, Ayurvedic scrubs gently remove old cells and help balance your doshas. Made with finely ground vegetable powders and herbs that are mixed with a small amount of liquid (see "Using the Right Scrub for Your Dosha," above), they are safe even for dry vata skin and sensitive pitta skin.

To Use Herbal Scrubs · Combine 1 tablespoon of each powdered ingredient and store in an airtight opaque container. To use, pour 1 to 2 teaspoons of the powder into the palm of your hand or a small dish; add enough liquid to form a paste. Apply to your face with your fingertips, and gently massage all over with small circular motions. Rinse off with cool water, and you are ready to apply a mask. If you wish to streamline your facial, you may leave the scrub on your face to use as a mask.

4. Fresh Fruit and Vegetable Mask

The fruit and vegetable masks suggested here are used for a variety of purposes. They deep clean by extracting dirt from pores. Because they are made from fresh edible ingredients, they nourish by providing vitamins and minerals. They rejuvenate tired, dull-looking skin by soothing, moisturizing, toning, stimulating circulation, and exfoliating. There's nothing like the right mask to brighten up your skin, leaving it cleaner, fresher, firmer, and younger looking. We provide two types of masks. The first is made of a base of pure fruits and vegetables; the second is made of powdered cosmetic purifying clay (available at health food stores and beauty supply shops). Try one of each type of mask and see which you prefer.

Fruit and Vegetable Masks. These masks are particularly gentle and soft; they contain vitamins and enzymes that are thought to feed your complexion, balance, tone, tighten, and improve your skin's circulation. The fruit acids contain natural, nontoxic, gentle forms of alpha-hydroxy acid, a popular substance in commercial skin "peels" because it removes dead cells (exfoliates). Choose the ingredients based on your dosha (see "Using the Right Fruit and Vegetable Mask for Your Dosha," page 130). Mash or blend the pulp with fork, potato masher, a mortar and pestle, or in a blender. Remember, since you are using pure natural ingredients, prepare the masks fresh and use immediately as they will spoil, as would any fresh food.

To help give the pulp more body and cohesion, so that it holds together on your face, add a little binder such as oat powder or cosmetic clay powder. Another method that will help keep the pulp in place is to make a cloth mask of cheesecloth or thin silk (use an old scarf). Cut an oval the size of your face, and remove circles for eyes, nostrils, and mouth. Place the cloth on your face and then apply the pulp on top of it so it soaks through to your skin. Wash the cloth mask well with mild soap and let dry between facials. Or you may dip the cloth in the juice of the fruit and then apply to your face. After applying the mask evenly to your face and throat, lie down

USING THE RIGHT FRUIT AND
❋ VEGETABLE MASK FOR YOUR DOSHA ❋

- *Vata Skin*: Use the pulp of one or more of the following: avocado, banana, pear, melon, nectarine, carrot.
- *Pitta Skin*: Use the pulp of one or more of the following: avocado, banana, cantaloupe, pineapple, peach, nectarine, zucchini.
- *Kapha Skin:* Use the pulp of one or more of the following: strawberry, pear, lemon (diluted half and half with water), papaya, cucumber, or to-mato. (Do not leave papaya on for more than five minutes.)
- *Dry or Mature Skin (all doshas):* Apply a pulp of cherries as a mask; you may add a little honey if you like.
- *Very Oily or Blemished Skin (all doshas):* Use the pulp of one or more of the following: apple, grape, tomato, or cabbage.

for fifteen to twenty minutes to allow the benefits to penetrate. Then rinse off with cool water.

Clay Masks. For these masks, clay is used as a base because clay tends to draw out impurities in the skin and refine the pores. Clay can also be a rich source of minerals. Adding the herbs and essential oils conveys the added benefit of balancing the doshas. Cosmetic purifying clay is available at health food stores; we prefer French green clay, which has a very fine texture. Refer to "Clay Masks According to Your Dosha," page 131 for the appropriate ingredients. Apply the paste evenly to your face and throat; lie down for fifteen to twenty minutes until it has dried, then rinse off with cool water.

5. Moisturize

After rinsing off the mask, moisturize your face as usual.

DAY TWO: PAMPER YOUR BODY

Today is the day you pamper your whole body. Believe it or not, every beauty treatment you give your face is also exquisitely pleasurable and ben-

❁ CLAY MASKS ACCORDING TO YOUR DOSHA ❁

- *Vata Skin:* Combine 6 teaspoons of clay; 2 teaspoons of either aloe vera juice or pure water; 1 teaspoon honey; 1 teaspoon of powdered licorice, chamomile, comfrey, rose, sandalwood, or orange peel and 3 drops of essential oil of rose, neroli, or chamomile.
- *Pitta Skin:* Combine 6 teaspoons of clay; 2 teaspoons of either aloe vera juice or pure water; 1 teaspoon honey; 1 teaspoon of powdered licorice, sandalwood, chamomile, clover, comfrey, fennel, lavender, or rose. And 3 drops essential oil of lavender, geranium, or sandalwood.
- *Kapha Skin:* Combine 5 teaspoons of clay; 1 teaspoon each of aloe vera juice, lemon juice, and honey; 1 teaspoon of powdered fennel, lavender, lemon balm, lemon peel, lemon verbena, rosemary, sandalwood, or dash-moola; and 3 drops of essential oil of juniper, bergamot, or cypress.
- *Very Oily or Blemished Skin*: Combine 6 teaspoons of clay; 3 teaspoons of honey; and 2 teaspoons of pure water. Pierce and add the contents of one 400 IU (international units) capsule of vitamin E, and one 10,000 IU capsule of vitamin A or beta-carotene.

eficial for your body. So today, treat every part of you as if it were as precious and as visible as your facial complexion. Simply follow the same steps (except for the steaming) as for Day One, using the same skin products. To review:

1. *Aromatic Oil Massage*: pamper yourself with a rich oil massage (Abhyanga) as directed in Step 5, using the massage oil suitable for your dosha. During the massage, pay particular attention to your feet and hands (see "A Special Treat for Your Hands and Feet," page 132). You may take a warm bath afterward, while the oil is still on your body.
2. *Herbal Scrub*: remove the oil and exfoliate with a chickpea flour paste enlivened with herbs. To allow the herbs to penetrate, leave the paste on your body and lie down for fifteen to twenty minutes. Because as turmeric will stain, use old sheets or towels to wrap yourself in. Rinse off in the shower.

A SPECIAL TREAT
❋ FOR YOUR HANDS AND FEET ❋

As part of your Once-a-Month Spa Program, give your hands and feet a soothing massage followed by a manicure and pedicure.

Hand Massage: After this pampering, your hands will be supple, graceful, and relaxed. Begin by applying warmed oil, suitable to your dosha. Work on one hand at a time, using the opposite hand. With your thumb, massage the ligaments on the back of your hand from the wrist to the webs between your fingers. Then massage the palm, working your way from the wrist up to the base of each finger. Massage each individual finger by grasping it between your thumb and index finger and working your way up to the fingertip. Pull each finger gently, rotate it, and squeeze the sides of the tip. Press the web between your thumb and index finger, as close to the juncture of the bones as possible. Do the other hand. Then vigorously rub your palms together until the friction creates heat. Rub each palm over the back of the other hand.

Foot Massage: To give a foot massage, begin by applying warmed oil, suitable to your dosha. Work on one foot at a time, with your ankle propped up on the thigh of your other leg. Massage the ankle, working the oil into the bones and gently squeezing the Achilles tendon between your thumb and forefinger. With your thumb, massage the ligaments on the top of your foot from the ankle to the webs between your toes. Then massage the sole of your foot, working your way from the heel up to the base of each toe, paying particular attention to the instep. Next, massage each individual toe by grasping it between your thumb and index finger and working your way out to the tip. Pull each toe gently, rotate it, and squeeze the sides of the tip. About one inch below the web, press the point between the tendon of your big toe and the adjacent toe. Then vigorously rub the top and sole of the foot until the friction creates heat. Cradle your foot in your hands for a moment before repeating the procedure with the other foot. Put on warm socks to help the oil penetrate your skin.

3. *Fresh Fruit and Vegetable Mask*: apply a fruit or vegetable mask all over your body to nourish, exfoliate, and rejuvenate.

4. *Moisturize*: use a base oil enriched with aromatic essential oils appropriate for your dosha.

❋ THE PROFESSIONAL SPA EXPERIENCE ❋

The word *panchakarma* comes from the Sanskrit words *pancha* meaning "five" and *karma* meaning "actions." This refers to the five pathways that are used to rid the body of poisons: the nose, the esophagus, stomach, bowels, and skin. If you decide to be treated at a panchakarma center, the purifying procedures can be quite an intense experience. However, they are performed with royal tender loving care and professionalism and are overseen by a doctor specializing in Ayurveda. The selected group of purification and lubrication techniques in this chapter are gentle, modified versions and can be safely and comfortably performed right in your own home.

INTERNAL SPA PROGRAM: LUBRICATION AND PURIFICATION

This aspect of the program consists of an at-home version of the lubricating, cleansing, and purification practices known in Ayurveda as panchakarma. These practices deeply relax and strengthen the whole system. They do this first and foremost by helping you rid your body of accumulated poisons from the air, water, and food. By ridding your body of this ama, your body can better absorb all those good nutrients you are providing with the Ayurvedic diet. Panchakarma also helps release toxic emotional stresses that can debilitate your nervous system. These practices have immense rejuvenative power—they improve cell activity and metabolism and revitalize all your tissues, your mind, and your spirit to stave off signs of premature aging and promote longevity.

When doing internal cleansing, remember that this program will be less jarring for your system if you have been living the healthy life described in Step 6: going to bed early and getting up early, spending calm and relaxed evenings, eating well, meditating, and doing yoga regularly. However, if you have been living a toxic, exhausting life, the first few times you follow this program may have a dramatic effect. You may experience almost a healing crisis because you are squeezing out an immense amount of poisons and emotional debris that is clogging your system. When I first tried these practices, I was drinking coffee, working very hard, I was exhausted. I had a lot of poisons to get rid of and as a result, I was evacuating my bowels a lot, which can be rather enervating. By the third or fourth time I did this program though, this was no longer the case, and the whole process was a breeze.

There are two parts to internal cleansing and purifying. Part One serves to mobilize ama, the accumulated toxins in your body so that the body is ready for Part Two, in which the actual deep internal cleansing takes place. Although these are milder versions of traditional panchakarma techniques, internal cleansing is still serious business. You need to plan for it. It's best if you use these practices in the morning and try to arrange your work schedule so that you have light workdays, especially during Part Two (Days 4, 5, and 6). Try to avoid scheduling important meetings, having deadlines for big projects, and so on. However, if your schedule is not flexible enough, just do the best you can and modify the program if you need to. *Precautions.* **Do not do this program if you have been diagnosed with a medical condition, such as diabetes, cancer, heart disease (unless you are under the care of an Ayurvedic physician); are pregnant, lactating, or within three months postdelivery; have poor appetite; have a fever; are obese; have an acute infection or inflammation; are menstruating. This program is not suitable for children**.

PART ONE: MOBILIZE AMA

The herbal and dietary measures of the first three days will prepare you for the deep internal cleansing of the last three days. If your digestion is generally fine, take the Oil and Water Elixir, which lubricates and hydrates your system. However, if you have digestive problems such as abdominal bloating, pain in your stomach after eating, gas, or constipation, then do the Ten-Day Ginger Treatment instead of the Elixir (plan to start then seven days earlier, so you finish on Day 3). You will also be eating Kicharee (recipe follows) during the first three days.

Days 1, 2, and 3

1. Oil and Water Elixir · The purpose of this is to lubricate and re-hydrate the dehydrated tissues inside your body so that the poisons they are

❀ TEN-DAY GINGER TREATMENT ❀

This special treatment lubricates your tissues and stokes your digestive fire. Mix together 8 teaspoons each of grated fresh gingerroot, brown sugar, and melted ghee (see ghee recipe, page 32). Store in your refrigerator, and each morning before breakfast, take the following amount. This remedy is surprisingly delicious, and the gingery, buttery, sugary feeling stays with you all day. (Note: vegans may substitute grape-seed oil for the ghee.)

Day 1:   ½ tsp.
Day 2:   1 tsp.
Day 3:   1½ tsp.
Day 4:   2 tsp.
Day 5:   2½ tsp.
Day 6:   2½ tsp.
Day 7:   2 tsp.
Day 8:   1½ tsp.
Day 9:   1 tsp.
Day 10: ½ tsp.

Precautions. Ginger can be too strong for some people's stomachs. Do not use this treatment if you have any severe stomach problems such as heartburn, unless you are under the care of an Ayurvedic physician.

holding onto will dissolve and slide out more easily. Boil the water for ten minutes to energize it, then let cool to just warm. Each of the three days, first thing upon arising, take one of the following:

Vata types. Take 1 tablespoon of olive oil mixed with 1 cup of boiled water. Follow this with a squeeze of fresh lime juice directly in your mouth.

Pitta types. Take 1 tablespoon of ghee (clarified butter; see recipe on page 32) mixed with 1 cup of boiled water. Follow this with a squeeze of fresh orange juice directly in your mouth.

Kapha types. Take 1 tablespoon of sunflower oil and ½ teaspoon of powdered ginger mixed with 1 cup of boiled water. Follow this with two capsules of cayenne taken with a cup of boiled water.

2. Dietary Detox · Eat only Kicharee for breakfast, lunch, and dinner (see recipe box page 137). You should also drink this spiced tea: combine ⅓ teaspoon each of powdered ginger, cinnamon, and cumin with 1 cup of water; bring to a boil and simmer for five minutes. Drink as much as you want of this delicious brew throughout the day, preferably plain, but you may add a little raw sugar if you need to or try stevia, a natural, calorie-free sweetener.

PART TWO: DEEP INTERNAL CLEANSING

The last three days consist of lubrication and purification techniques.

Days 4, 5, and 6:

1. Oil Massage · Before you can eliminate toxins, you need to condition and lubricate your body so that the toxins can be released. In Ayurveda, this means oiling your body with massage. This massage is similar to the daily Abhyanga technique described in Step 5; it should take about twenty minutes or so, if you go slowly and deliberately and pay loving attention to every part of your body. Vata types use sesame or almond oil. Pitta types use coconut or sunflower oil. Kaphas use mustard seed oil.

1. Follow the general instructions for Abhyanga (see page 90), making long up and down strokes on the long bones of your arms and legs and circular motions on your joint. Pay a lot of attention to your third eye—the point on your forehead between your eyes. Massage deeply into your skull at this point and all over your forehead.

2. For purification purposes, pour a few drops of warmed oil in your ears and massage the outer ear canal gently with the tip of your pinky finger. Massage the outer ear and pull down gently on your earlobes. Then insert a small ball of cotton to retain the oil in your ears for the duration of the massage and the steam treatment that follows.

3. Insert a small amount of oil into your navel and massage it into the abdominal area in a circular clockwise direction: massaging first your ascending colon going up the right side of your abdomen, then across the transverse colon right to left, then down your left abdo-

❉ KICHAREE ❉

Kicharee is a medicinal meal consisting of rice, lentils, herbs, spices, and vegetables. It was used traditionally to bring very sick people back to health. We recommend it before and during the monthly program, but you can eat this delicious, soothing dish any time you are feeling overtaxed or wish to get off the junk food bandwagon. It is easily digestible, high in protein, pure and wholesome and wonderfully comforting and satisfying.

> ¼ tsp. cumin seeds
> 2 T. ghee or sunflower oil
> 3 bay leaves
> ½ tsp. turmeric
> 1 tsp. oregano
> 1 stick kombu (seaweed)
> 1 tsp. grated fresh ginger
> ½ cup basmati rice
> ¼ cup split mung dahl (lentils)
> 4 to 6 cups water
> 3 cups diced fresh vegetables such as carrots, zucchini, squash, parsnips.

Wash the lentils and rice until the water runs clear. Warm the ghee in a medium saucepan; add the cumin, bay, coriander, and oregano. Brown slightly until their aroma is released. Stir in turmeric, rice, and dahl. Add water, salt, kombu, and ginger. Simmer, covered, over medium heat for about a half an hour, or until lentils and rice are soft. Add vegetables and cook ten to fifteen minutes, or until tender.

men to massage the descending colon, and back across your lower abdomen from left to right. Work slowly, and make loving, deliberate circles, exerting firm pressure to stimulate your digestive tract.

4. Massage your chest from the outside toward the inside, then the inside toward the outside, and massage from the clavicle (collarbone) down toward the heart. When working on your rib cage, exhale before massaging.

5. As you work on your face, massage your jaw with upward stokes and open your mouth as you massage your temples.

6. Finally, open your mouth and press the center of your palate with the tip of your thumb; then press the top of your skull. Hold each of these points for about fifteen seconds. These marma points serve to stimulate brain chemistry regulation. If it feels good to you and you feel a rush of clarity, you can do this again later in the evening.

Now your tissues are wonderfully soft and lubricated. Do not shower or bathe immediately. Rest quietly for a few minutes before going on to the Sweat Bath.

2. Sweat Bath · While your body is still oiled, you heat your body in a steam box, which causes you to sweat. Sweating is wonderfully relaxing. The internal heat helps liquify ama so that it can be more easily and completely eliminated through digestion and sweating. Sweating also melts and helps you get rid of hardened, crystalized emotions. In India, men traditionally performed sweating rituals to rid themselves of the poison emotions they brought back with them from wars. Native Americans also used sweat lodges to purify their bodies and spirits.

According to Ayurveda, it is harmful to subject your head to heat, so a sauna or steam room will not work. Therefore you will need to purchase a sweatbox, which is like a one-person stream room, but one that leaves your head free. I use a sweatbox from Sears, which costs only $150 and comes with a comfortable seat, taking up only about the same space as a home computer. At first, my patients balk at the expense. But when they compare the cost of a sweatbox with the cost of a single day at a professional spa (several hundred dollars), they soon stop their grumbling.

To use the sweatbox:

1. Sit comfortably, and place a washcloth dipped in cool water on your forehead. Wrap a towel around your neck to seal in the heat. Remain for ten minutes.
2. Get out of the sweatbox, and remove the oil with a paste of chickpea flour and water. Simply apply the paste to your whole body and massage well.
3. Then rinse off in the shower with lukewarm water.
4. Follow this with meditation, breathing exercises, and light yoga.

Have Kicharee for dinner, spend a quiet evening, and then go to bed early.

When you go through purification—even this milder at-home version—you'll feel much more in charge, more alive. Your skin will glow, your eyes will sparkle, and you will feel great. There will be less mystery to your inner workings, and you will see the incredible results. For me, this is one of the most powerful and rewarding things about helping people though this process—they start to feel really connected to their bodies. And with that connection comes a greater ease, grace, and inner and outer beauty.

The Once-a-Month Spa Program is a powerful tool and will give you incredible results. It will also pave the way for the deeper cleansing and remarkable rejuvenation possible when you undertake Step 8, which is a more intense version of panchakarma.

STEP 8

Seasonal Purification Program

THE SEASONAL PURIFICATION PROGRAM IS DESIGNED TO BUILD on the daily and monthly routines in Steps 6 and 7. The earlier steps are in themselves cleansing and revitalizing, but it takes the more rigorous and lengthy program we provide in this chapter to remove stubborn, deep-seated impurities and toxins that are dulling your skin and hair and making it difficult to control your weight.

In Ayurveda the transitional time between seasons is traditionally the time for personal renewal. From the Ayurvedic point of view this makes sense because all year, in a never-ending cycle, nature shifts from old energy to new energy. Nature's rhythms bring you along whether you are ready or not and unless you take action, you will be dragging the energy from one season to the next, creating stress and strain. Ayurveda helps you move the transitional process along, making you more resilient and more in tune with the rhythms of nature. What better way to help ease you through the transition from season to season than treating yourself to a two-week program designed to clear out the dust and the cobwebs, to make sure your body's furnace, air-conditioning, electricity, and garbage disposal are all working properly?

The stepped-up version of panchakarma is similar to the process introduced in Step 7, but it is more intense and of longer duration. Admittedly, this level of intensity is not for everyone—it's for those who are die-hard experienced adherents of Ayurveda who have prepared themselves by following Step 6, the Daily Spa Program for several months and who have gone through Step 7 , the Once-a-Month Spa Program at least twice. However, if you are not willing or able to do both the monthly program and the seasonal program, the seasonal program takes precedence because the seasonal influences are so strong.

You could undergo similar treatments at a spa for hundreds of dollars a day—or you could do our safe, streamlined version in the privacy of your own home at a fraction of the cost. You, too, can enjoy the centuries-old pleasure of rejuvenation, maintain and restore health and beauty, create for yourself inner strength and joy, free up your innate intelligence, cultivate your unique radiance, and possibly extend your youthfulness and your life.

Timing and Preparation

Follow this program four times a year, at the change of the seasons. In the United States this means the third week in:

- March (when winter changes to spring)
- June (when spring changes to summer)
- September (when summer changes to fall)
- December (when fall changes to winter)

Panchakarma is a powerful process, and it requires your respect. You need to set aside time, plan for it, mark it in your calendar as if you were going away on vacation. It is hard work for your body and mind to do double duty as both giver and recipient. You are both housecleaner and house during an intense cleanup that removes all the debris that has accumulated in the past three months.

The seasonal program begins with a ten-day preparation period that is followed by four days of strenuous cleansing practices. Unless otherwise specified, aim to perform the procedures in the morning, in sequence. However, if your schedule does not allow this, you may do some or all of the practices at night. Try to arrange your schedule so that you have lighter workdays during the four days of strenuous cleansing. Take it easy at home, too—do light chores, quiet social activities, gentle yoga, and a modified exercise program. Try to meditate twice a day, and spend some of your time contemplating, taking stock, and planning for the upcoming season.

If you feel some new sensations during this program, don't be afraid or get upset. Embrace these sensations—that is what this program is all about: out with the old, make room for the new. Simply breathe your way through the experience, filling your body with new air and new life and expelling the old. When you meditate, let go of useless outmoded thoughts and thought patterns. During yoga get to know yourself and let your physical self expand, grow, and open up to new possibilities. As long as we have a body, we must cherish it and care for it. Our inner beauty grows with this love.

Precautions. **Do not do this program if you are fearful or hesitant about undergoing an intense physical and emotional experience; stay with the monthly program until you are physically and mentally stronger. Do not do this program if you have been diagnosed with a medical condition, such as diabetes, cancer, heart disease (unless you are under the care of an Ayurvedic physician); are pregnant, lactating, or within three months postdelivery; have a poor appetite; have a fever; are obese; have an acute infection or inflammation; are menstruating. You should not do the oil enema if you have hemorrhoids. This program is not suitable for children.**

PREPARING YOUR MIND AND BODY

DAYS 1–10: JUMP-START CLEANSING

Before you begin the deep-cleansing portion of the program, prepare your mind and body.

1. Ten-Day Ginger Treatment

Do the Ten-Day Ginger Treatment (see page 135) to stimulate agni, your digestive fire, and begin the purification process.

2. Five-Day Dietary Detox

For Days 6 through 10, eliminate all alcohol, caffeine, smoke, refined sugars and grains, drugs, meat, and dairy to reduce the burden of toxic substances. Eat as follows:

- *Breakfast*: Eat a light breakfast of fruit, oatmeal, and vata tea.
- *Lunch*: Eat a bowl of Kicharee (see recipe, page 137).
- *Dinner*: Have a clear broth and a generous amount of plain cooked vegetables. Squash, yams, and steamed bitter greens are recommended.
- Each day drink four quarts of hot water with lemon juice to taste.

CLEANSING YOUR MIND AND BODY

DAY 11

1. Licorice Tea

Drink three glasses of warm licorice tea first thing in the morning. This may cause vomiting in some people; don't worry—this is part of the purification process and helps reduce kapha in your body.

2. Zesty Herbal Wake-Up

Combine in a blender 1 teaspoon of lime juice, a 1-inch piece of fresh peeled chopped ginger, ¼ teaspoon sea salt, ¼ teaspoon cayenne pepper, a handful of fresh cilantro, and ½ cup water. Blend until smooth and drink. This warms the stomach and helps burn off the ama. Your stomach should not feel a burning sensation, but your throat may. If this occurs, take ½ teaspoon of honey mixed with ½ teaspoon of shatavari to soothe it.

3. Oil Massage

Follow the directions for the lubricating oil massage on page 131 in Step 7. If you like, you may also massage a small amount of mustard oil into your chest. This will help clean out any mucus you may have accumulated in your lungs. You might spit up mucus, even though you are not ill, as I did the first time I did this practice. The mucus represents clogged kapha and stuck thoughts.

4. Sesame Oil Gargle and Nasaya

Gargle with sesame oil and sniff two to three drops of sesame oil into your nose, a practice called Nasaya, lubrication of nasal passages. You may do a more intense version of Nasaya, as follows, which is more effective and is more appropriate as part of a seasonal program. You can do this yourself, but we recommend you have a helper.

1. Grate some fresh ginger and catch the juice in an eye dropper.
2. Lie down on your back and have your helper put a drop of the juice in each nostril. Inhale slightly—and be ready for your nasal passages to explode in a five-alarm fire. The burning will last a few seconds and then vanish completely.
3. Immediately have your helper put a drop of sesame oil in each nostril and inhale (use warm ghee for pittas)—this will completely calm any residual stinging sensation or agitation you may feel.

7. Sweat Bath

Follow the instructions in Step 7 for taking a sweat bath (page 138). If you like, you may first apply a sandalwood paste (powdered sandalwood mixed with water) to your face. Sit in the steam for no more than ten minutes. Relax for a few minutes after the steam, remove the oil with a paste made of chickpea powder and water, and shower in lukewarm water.

8. Food Guidelines

Eat a small bowl of Kicharee for breakfast and dinner (see recipe, page 137), with a larger one for lunch.

9. Anti-Aging Formula

Before going to bed, take ½ teaspoon each of triphala and ghee mixed with 1 teaspoon of honey with warm water. This is a gentle rejuvenating Anti-aging Herbal Formula.

DAY 12

1. Oil Massage

Give yourself a lubricating oil massage as for Day 11.

2. Sweat Bath

Give yourself a sweat bath as for Day 11.

3. Food Guidelines

Eat Kicharee for breakfast, lunch, and dinner.
Drink licorice tea throughout the day.

4. Anti-Aging Formula

Before going to bed, take ½ teaspoon each of triphala and ghee mixed
with 1 teaspoon of honey with warm water.

5. Minimassage

Place a small amount of oil in your navel and massage your abdomen;
also give your ears and your feet an oil massage (for instructions of giving
a foot massage, see page 132). Vatas use sesame oil, pittas use coconut oil,
and kaphas use mustard oil.

DAY 13

1. Zesty Herbal Wake-Up

First thing in the morning, prepare and drink the lime juice, ginger,
sea salt, cayenne pepper, cilantro drink as for Day 11.

❋ THE TRADITION OF SHIRODARA ❋

Traditionally, Shirodara involves pouring a steady stream of warm oil on the third eye of your forehead for thirty minutes. Ayurveda considers the forehead to be the center of thought, the place in the brain where higher states of thoughts and emotions are processed. Shirodara deeply relaxes the cranial muscles so that any stress that is locked into the tissues slips away.

---

2. Shirodara (Shir-oh-DA-rah)

Shirodara (see "The Tradition of Shirodara," above) requires specialized equipment and is most effective when done professionally. However, you can practice an at-home version using an oil compress. To do Shirodara:

1. Take a soft cotton cloth such as a washcloth and fold it into thirds, forming a long rectangle. Bring the ends of the rectangle together, folding it in half crosswise.
2. Dip this center fold into warmed sesame oil, thoroughly saturating that part of the cloth but leaving the ends dry.
3. Lie down in a warm, quiet, comfortable place and place the compress on your forehead, with the oil-soaked portion over your third eye. Place another cloth or folded towel over the compress to keep the heat in. Relax for ten minutes, with your eyes closed.

3. Oil Massage

Do the lubricating oil massage as for Day 11.

4. Food Guidelines

Eat Kicharee for breakfast, lunch, and dinner.
Drink as much fennel tea as you like throughout the day.
Take 1 cup of warm milk mixed with 1 teaspoon of ghee at midday.

You may also eat small amounts of raisins, steamed greens, broccoli, and beets.

5. Herbal Tea Laxative

Before going to bed, take ½ teaspoon of triphala mixed with 1 cup of warm water. This acts as a mild laxative, which will help evacuate your bowels tomorrow and enhance the elimination of toxins and old energy.

6. Anti-Aging Formula

Before going to bed, take ½ teaspoon each of triphala and ghee mixed with 1 teaspoon of honey with warm water.

DAY 14

1. Oil Massage

Do the lubricating oil massage as for Day 11.

2. Nasaya

Do either the sesame oil or ginger Nasaya as for Day 11.

3. Sweat Bath

Give yourself a sweat bath as for Day 11.

4. Basti

After the previous treatments your body will be ready to release the deep toxins that are lodged in the tissues. To facilitate this process, you do a treatment called Basti (see "About Basti" on page 149). Basti is a procedure that does not appeal to many people at first thought. But after employing the method or having it done at a spa, most people enjoy a great feeling of well-being and become enthusiastic advocates. Doing it at home is simple.

❋ ABOUT BASTI ❋

It is said in the ancient Ayurvedic texts that this practice is so powerful that it prevents 70 percent of all disease. Basti, the introduction of oil into the rectum, is not the same as a water enema. Water enemas are designed solely to evacuate your colon, but they have a tendency to dry out the mucus membranes. Oil Basti may cause you to have a bowel movement—or several, during the course of the day. This can be beneficial, but it is not the true or most important purpose of this practice. Rather, basti is designed to lubricate, purify, and rejuvenate the walls of the colon and nourish the entire body. Basti is an important practice because in Ayurveda, your colon is a bridge to all the organs of your body.

---

1. Buy a rectal bulb in the drugstore. Fill with 1 cup of warmed oil and a little warm water. Vatas and pittas use sesame oil; kaphas use sunflower oil.
2. Administer as you would a water enema.
3. Basti may or may not cause you to evacuate your bowels. Because this is a powerful treatment, the aftereffects vary from person to person; it is safest to rest for twenty minutes after the basti and to wear an absorbent pad because as the day wears on leaking of oil can occur. Do not do strenuous exercise or work today; rest as much as possible and ease your way into moderate activity.

Precaution. **Do not do basti if you are pregnant, or may be pregnant, or if you have a bowel or rectum disorder.**

5. *Food Guidelines*

Eat Kicharee for breakfast, lunch, and dinner.
Drink as much fennel tea as you like throughout the day.
Take 1 cup of warm milk mixed with 1 teaspoon of ghee at midday.
You may also eat small amounts of raisins, steamed greens, broccoli, and beets.

6. *Anti-Aging Formula*

Before bed, take ½ teaspoon each of triphala and ghee mixed with 1 teaspoon of honey with warm water.

EASING BACK INTO YOUR NORMAL ROUTINE

Gradually return to the Daily Spa Routine in Step 7. For the next three days, have a normal breakfast, eat Kicharee for lunch and soup and salad for dinner. Avoid heavy foods, but if you must have meat, avoid red meat and opt for small amounts of well-cooked fish or chicken. Try to rest as much as possible, get some sun in the morning or late afternoon every day, take long easy walks, and be in silence to absorb and appreciate the effects of panchakarma.

Take a *rasayana* following your treatment. A rasayana is a collection of herbs that nourish and rejuvenate; they work particularly powerfully after your body has been prepared by panchakarma. Take the rasayana in warm water in the morning and evening for the three days following the seasonal program. Then take it just once a day in the morning for the next month.

- Vata: take ½ teaspoon ashwagandha.
- Pitta: take ½ teaspoon shatavari.
- Kapha: take ¼ teaspoon each of trikatu and ashwagandha.

Enhancing the Program

To get the most out of the Seasonal Purification Spa Program, keep these pointers in mind:

- If possible make this a time for doing additional or extended meditation and breathing exercises. Chant if you like, or sing. Do gentle yoga, progressing through the postures slowly and deliberately, paying special attention to your breathing.
- Take a break from your usual exercise program; instead, take slow

walks in nature, or an easy swim. Vatas should absolutely avoid any strenuous exercise at this time. Pittas can do a somewhat strenuous activity, but not competitive. If you are kapha, you may hike uphill and break a sweat.

- Eat light, simple, easily digested foods such as Kicharee throughout the six days of the program. At least avoid heavy breads, meat, or rich sauces.
- Avoid TV, loud music, and get enough rest and sleep.
- Take a break from your usual chores and focus on nurturing, non-stress-provoking activities such as working in the garden, cleaning out an old closet, straightening out a photo album or scrapbook—something that will give you a sense of accomplishment.
- Sit in a quiet place where you will not be interrupted, get out your organizer or calendar, and do your planning for the next month. Take advantage of the literal and symbolic clean start this practice will give you, and consider the big picture for the coming month—what do you want to accomplish?
- Consciously pay attention to yourself and to this program. Think about how clean you will feel, how much strength and clarity you will gain. Imagine how effortless it will be for you to complete your goals because you are taking the time out now to perform the tasks needed to purify, rejuvenate, restore you body so you have what it takes to complete the challenges you create for yourself.

It takes willpower to make the decision to purify and change your life. At first panchakarma—even in this relatively mild form—may be difficult or somewhat uncomfortable because you are going against your usual routine, paying attention to yourself, and accelerating the removal of deep-seated toxins. But after that, the decision to take care of and nurture yourself becomes effortless. Each time you do this program, it should be less fatiguing and less difficult. As your body gets used to the program, it is less stressed and learning a new way to be, to feel, and it becomes cleaner, purer. You will emerge stronger, and the next time you do it you will have so much determination, it's almost magical.

Because my patients are learning something completely different, at first I sometimes hear them complain that it seems "too different" or "weird." But once they have made the commitment and gone through the procedures, I hear them say "Wow! I felt so much more grounded and energized for weeks afterward! During panchakarma I felt in control of my life; it did so much for my health. I felt proud that I was able to accomplish it." In completing the Seasonal Purification Program, you deserve to be proud of yourself, too, and in a strong and motivated position to progress to the next step—controlling your weight.

STEP 9

Effortless Weight Control Program

*E*VEN MORE THAN HAVING FLAWLESS SKIN AND SHINY HAIR, MY patients want to be their ideal weight. Many of my new patients come to me feeling depressed and dejected about their weight—almost to the point of giving up ever trying to lose weight. But after following the Ayurvedic weight control practices I recommend, those with extra pounds invariably are pleasantly surprised to find the excess weight has come off naturally. Those rare individuals who could use a few more pounds are also amazed to see themselves filling out just as they had always wanted. The same can happen to you.

The beauty-enhancing daily, monthly, and seasonal spa programs in Steps 6, 7, and 8 will help you balance your doshas, establish good eating habits, and clear out accumulated toxins that clog your system. If you have a mild weight problem, they may be all you need to achieve your ideal weight. But if your doshas are tipped too much off balance or if your excess weight stubbornly refuses to budge, you will need to follow those steps with a program designed specifically to restore your ideal weight. In this case, the spa programs are still important because they set the stage for effortless weight loss by priming your mind and body to absorb the nutrients you need and clearing the way for your system to shed excess pounds.

You won't find a "diet" in this chapter. Rather, you'll find a truly holistic weight control program, with individualized weight control plans that include satisfying amounts of tasty foods that are "friendly" to your body type so that you feel satisfied rather than deprived. You'll never look haggard, drawn, or dried out, for the excess weight falls off naturally.

We begin by revealing the secret to weight control from the Ayurvedic point of view. We then show you how you can put these principles to use by following our specific advice for each of the doshas, including the use of herbs and spices that miraculously make the pounds melt away. Then we supply general practices that apply to all the doshas. Next, we provide a section of dealing with special issues surrounding weight and body shape: abdominal bloating, cellulite, food cravings, and water retention. Because most people in this country want to lose weight, this chapter focuses primarily on that issue. However, for those who need to gain weight, we have devoted the last section of this chapter to that problem.

Whether you weigh just a few more pounds than you'd like to or a few less, or whether your weight problem is more significant than that—Ayurveda can help put you back on track effortlessly because by using Ayurvedic techniques you are working with your natural body type and its needs.

THE SECRET TO WEIGHT CONTROL

Ayurveda considers overweight and underweight to be signs that your doshas are out of balance. Although of course *how much* you eat is a factor, it is only half the story. The other half is how well the food you eat is absorbed and metabolized. Whether you want to lose or gain weight, the strategy in Ayurveda weight control is to permanently reset your body-mind's ability to regulate itself by enhancing your digestive fires, regulating the storage of energy and fat, and calming your nervous system, which orchestrates everything.

The Role of Digestion and Metabolism

Good digestion is the key to health, beauty, and achieving your ideal weight. It is the path that nature created for you to transform substances from your environment into your physical body. Will you transform it into lean tissue or fat? Will what you eat be available to rebuild the cells in your body? Will it go where it is needed, or will it sit there like a lump?

Poor digestion and metabolism creates ama, accumulated toxins and waste products. Excess ama clogs your channels, making you feel lethargic, encouraging you to eat erratically and impulsively, turning into excess weight, and making it difficult for you to lose weight. If you tend to overweight, improving your digestion will enable you to metabolize more food without gaining weight.

How the Doshas Influence Weight

Overweight is usually a function of kapha, the dosha that is composed of water and earth. When this dosha is imbalanced, the heavy characteristics of the elements of earth and water become exaggerated. Naturally, an excess of kapha most strongly affects people with predominantly kapha-type constitutions. But everyone consists of some kapha and once your fat metabolism becomes out of balance, the pounds either pile up (if the metabolism is slow) or they fall off (if the metabolism is fast). The enzymes in your system, which are the little engines that break down ingested food and help convert to high octane fuel, get diminished or blocked. Fat metabolism stops and fat accumulates and clogs up your system.

However, weight problems don't belong only to kapha types. That's because all the doshas are involved in digestion and metabolism. Vata is like the nervous system, and the metaphor for vata is the wind. Pitta is the digestive system, and the metaphor is fire; kapha is lymph and fat and, as stated earlier, the metaphor is earth and water. Overweight occurs when the wind either blows the fire out or aggravates it. If the wind blows it out because the body is locked into the anxiety-alarm state, the digestive juices are not secreted. The food doesn't get broken down and your body can't use it, so your body is fooled into thinking it's hungry and starving, so you eat more and more even though the body may be actually forty to fifty pounds overweight. On the other hand, if the overwrought vata fans the fire and increases it, earth and water tries to put the fire out, which translates into more fat and fluid.

What This Means for Your Dosha

Kapha types are born with a natural tendency to gain weight easily and lose it with difficulty, even when they are in balance. Combined with a naturally full-fleshed body type and a natural aversion to exercise, this tendency means that overweight is often a chronic battle for kaphas. When kaphas are overweight, they tend to be very heavy, sluggish, lethargic, and depressed.

Pitta types usually have no problem with weight, but they can gain weight if their digestive fire is too low because they have burned themselves out. They don't process food (or emotions) properly, and this results in weight gain. When pittas are overweight, they tend to be red-faced, retain water, look bloated and puffy, and feel agitated and irritable.

Vata types usually weigh less than they would like. When vata is imbalanced, the components of the nervous system, the pituitary, the thyroid, and the hypothalamus become overwhelmed or jammed. The neuroelectrical circuits that are the expression of vata energy become out of balance, and the system cannot absorb nutrients. However, even vata types can become overweight when imbalanced, if they attempt to calm and lubricate their over-stimulated and dry nervous systems with too many sweet, oily foods. In this way, vatas can gain weight during times of extreme anxiety and nervousness.

As a hard-driving pitta, I have always had a slight weight problem myself. Thanks to Ayurveda, I now know why, and I know what to do about it. I am naturally intense, and the intensity of working as a doctor, seeing thirty and sometimes forty patients a day one-on-one and then giving lectures and teaching workshops keeps my pitta aggravated. With these influences, it's difficult for me to stay in balance, and I must constantly work at it. But when my doctoring and my commitment to communicating and educating people don't get in the way, when I'm eating Kicheree, eating ghee, doing my nature walks, I drop 3 to 4 pounds effortlessly.

Before You Begin

Before embarking upon this program ask yourself: what can I realistically achieve, given my intrinsic body type? Understanding your body in Ayurvedic terms, which acknowledges that there are distinct body types with their own characteristics, is a wonderfully freeing experience. It not only relieves you of the burden of trying to look like someone else—some ideal figure sold to you by the media—but it also teaches you to appreciate your own unique characteristics for what they are—beautiful, or with the potential to be beautiful. Ayurveda recognizes that people are individuals. We can't all look the same. Nor would we want to because each body type has its own type of beauty when it is in balance.

Vata. Vata bodies naturally tend to be extreme—thin and delicately petite or elegantly tall. They have fine bones with narrow hips and shoulders or narrow hips and wide shoulders or the other way around. Most have long, slender, graceful limbs and fingers. Vatas can be strikingly sinewy or a bit soft—even flabby. Many of our physical role models are vatas or have starved themselves into looking like vatas.

Pitta. The typical pitta body is right in the middle, of medium build, somewhat athletic, with medium bone structure and height. Everything is well proportioned—shoulders, hips, limbs, fingers, toes, and medium-sized breasts. They tend to have nicely toned muscles and firm flesh. The well-toned, strong, self-assured, energetic aerobicized body is typically pitta.

Kapha. Kapha is the solid, heavy body type. They are strong and large, with abundant flesh and musculature. They have big bones and a broad frame with wide hips and shoulders and large, heavy breasts. Medium in height, they have well-proportioned limbs. The kapha body tends to overweight, but a balanced kapha is strong, voluptuous, sensual, and comforting. This is the least popular body type in our culture, but is worshipped as earth mother in other cultures.

If you are a vata you will never look like a pitta, and if you are a kapha you will never look like a vata—try as you may. However, a vata doesn't have to be painfully thin; nor does a kapha necessarily give up and resign herself to overweight. When you are in balance, you modify the extreme tendencies of your dosha. So a vata can be slender and elegant without being emaciated; a kapha can be voluptuous without being fat.

EATING GUIDELINES FOR YOUR DOSHA

The most effective weight control program is one that is tailored to your dosha; it is also the most effortless because it is going along with your essential nature, not against it. What is miraculously effective for you could be the worst strategy for your best friend, sister, or mother. So our eating plans are tailored to each dosha and consist of a daily eating pattern for breakfast lunch and dinner, followed by advice on foods, spices, and herbal formulas for each dosha.

Daily Eating Pattern

With this eating plan, there are no complicated menus to follow. Simply eat breakfast, lunch, and dinner while choosing foods appropriate for your dosha (see "Step 2: Nourishing Your Body"). As you select your foods, deemphasize foods high in fat, sugar, and calories, and include more foods high in fiber and nutrients and low in fat and calories. This means adding more vegetables, fruits, grains, and beans or lentils, and reducing the amount of oils, fried foods, pastries, cookies, and candy. Avoid prepared foods in general, because they often contain high amounts of refined sugar and flour as well as fats and additives that help keep the food fresh and palatable but aren't really needed for flavor or nutrition.

With its emphasis on whole fresh vegetables, grains, beans, and fruits, the Ayurvedic way of eating is already naturally low in fat and high in filling fiber, so it's hard to go wrong. This is not a radical or difficult way of eating, either. A diet based on vegetables is recommended by major public health agencies, such as the American Cancer Society. Research conducted by this organization found that people who eat four or more servings of meat per week were more likely to gain weight. But the more vegetables they ate, the less likely they were to gain. Earlier studies show that people who switch to eating vegetarian cuisine lose an average of 10 percent of their body weight.

Breakfast:

Ayurveda does not believe that you must eat a hearty breakfast.

- Kaphas may skip breakfast altogether and just have a cup of spiced herbal kapha tea and perhaps a piece of fresh, juicy fruit.
- Pittas and vatas can have a small bowl of whole grain cereal and milk, such as creamy oatmeal made with almond milk and spiced with churna.

Lunch:

This is should be your biggest meal of the day because this is the time when food is most digestible and least likely to create ama.

- Kaphas should eat a spicy dish such as curried vegetables (avoid root vegetables because they are heavy) made with aromatic Indian spices and served over steamed basmati rice; or vegetarian black bean chili.
- Pittas may have a hearty sandwich of grilled chicken or fish or marinated tofu with avocado and sprouts on whole grain bread with a vegetable salad on the side.
- Vatas should have a warming and hearty vegetable soup made with red lentils, split mung beans, or aduki beans. Take sweet lassi with your lunch daily. Prepare this delicious beverage by blending 6 ounces of water with 2 ounces of plain yogurt. Sweeten with raw unrefined sugar to taste.

Dinner:

This meal should be light and emphasize carbohydrates so that it is easily digested and helps you calm down for the evening and sleep soundly. The lentil dish known as Kicharee (see recipe page 137) is appropriate for all doshas. Alternatively:

- Kaphas can have a leafy vegetable salad with rice cakes or a corn tortilla with a spicy bean spread.

- Pittas start with a bitter melon soup followed by a medley of sautéed bitter greens, vegetables, and beans over basmati rice.
- Vatas may eat a vegetable or bean casserole with nutty whole grain bread or a pasta such as vegetarian lasagna.

Snacks:

Fresh fruit (eaten alone) is a good daytime snack; warmed spiced milk is an excellent nightcap. You may also drink as much herbal tea as you wish with meals or throughout the day. Each night around 7 P.M. vatas should eat a handful of sesame seeds and raisins.

Herbal and Spice Therapy for Kaphas

1. Pungent, bitter, and astringent spices kick kapha into high gear. Eat cayenne pepper and spicy herbs at least three times a week. These are found in many foods and spices—you can't eat too much ginger in particular—as well as the spring churna (a combination of herbs and spices; see page 63), which you can sprinkle on your food every day.
2. Drinking the following peppy concoction will burn the pounds away but admittedly is only for the stout at heart: mix the juice of five large slices of fresh pineapple with the juice of two slices of hot peppers, pimentos, or paprika.
3. Grate fresh ginger; add a little lemon and salt. Eat this right before your biggest meal, preferably at lunch.
4. You may also take triphala guggulu, a compound made from a resin of guggul, which is related to myrrh. It scrapes the fat off the inner lining of the entire digestive tract. Take ¼ teaspoon in warm water with 1 teaspoon of honey. Take two to three times a day if you are more than 20 pounds overweight.
5. Also try this herbal remedy: mix one part each of turmeric, triphala, trikatu, with two parts honey; take ⅛ teaspoon once a day, with ½ cup warm water.
6. The taste of this herbal combination admittedly leaves something to be desired, but the unpleasantness is worth it because it really works wonders. Combine 1 part each of the Ayurvedic herbs trikatu, chi-

trak, and kukti; take ½ teaspoon with a mouthful of warm water, swish around your mouth, and swallow. Take this once a day if you are twenty pounds overweight or less; take twice a day if you are more than twenty pounds overweight. Take between the hours of 6 to 10 A.M. or P.M.

Other Tips for Kaphas:

1. Warm, spicy aromas help stimulate kapha to burn up fat, so use eucalyptus, pine, musk, and sage aromatherapy.
2. The color red is recommended to stimulate sluggish kapha.
3. Daily dry massage (Garshana, page 92) using a silk glove is stimulating. You may also make an herbal paste of 1 part millet and ½ part each of the herbs dashmoola and bala mixed with a little spring water. Rub this vigorously onto your skin wherever you have fatty deposits; then rinse.

Herbal and Spice Therapy for Vatas

1. Sweet, sour, and salty tastes such as fennel, coriander, cumin, dill, salt, lemon, saffron, turmeric, ajwain, and those found in the spring churna (a combination of herbs and spices, see page 63).
2. Combine 1 teaspoon each of vidanga, chitrak, and kukti. Take ⅛ to ½ teaspoon daily, three to six times a day—the dosage and frequency depend on the severity of the problem. Mix with honey and warm water. This helps remove and prevent ama, improve digestion, enhance food absorption, and control appetite. Take between 2 and 6 A.M. or P.M.

Other Tips for Vatas

1. Essential oils with sweet warm aromas help calm vata and your nervous system, so choose jasmine, clove, rose, cinnamon, and orange scents for your aromatherapy. You may also add three drops of rose aromatherapy oil to two teaspoons of sesame or almond oil; apply this to your wrist and to the back of the head where the skull meets the neck bones (occipital ridge).
2. Daily full-body oil massage (Abhyanga, page 90) is essential for calming vata.

Herbal and Spice Therapy for Pittas

1. Bitter, pungent, and astringent herbs and spices are balancing for you, but the most important pitta taste is bitter. Bitter is the antidote for eliminating heat in the body. It is a difficult taste for many people of European descent; however, it is extremely important because pitta is a common body type amongst European descendants. Asian, African, and Mediterranean descendants also have pitta types, but bitter taste is well integrated into those traditional cooking preparations. Bitter, pungent, and astringent herbs and spices are found in the summer churna (a combination of herbs and spices, see page 63).
2. Take ½ teaspoon cumin and ½ teaspoon of coriander and soak in two cups of water overnight. Drink throughout the next day.
3. Milk is an important food for pittas, specifically small amounts of cooked milk with cumin, saffron, or fennel.
4. Rose ghee is particularly beneficial for pittas who are overweight. Place a layer of fragrant rose petals in a wide-mouthed glass container. Cover with a layer of ghee. Repeat this process three or four times, alternately layering the rose petals and the ghee. Leave overnight and in the morning remove the petals before using in cooking.
5. Combine 1 part each of brahmi, chitrak, and kukti. Take ½ teaspoon in warm water, once a day, between 10 A.M. to 2 P.M. only.
6. Take two to four tablets of Kaishore guggulu, per day.

Other Tips for Pittas

1. Essential oils with sweet cool aromas help stabilize vata, so choose honeysuckle, mint, and jasmine scents for your aromatherapy.
2. To stimulate and purify, give yourself a ten-minute Garshana (dry) massage every morning, using a silk glove (see page 92).
3. Try to avoid anger and irritability; do not eat when you are under emotional stress or are angry. Pittas may chronically overeat as a way of turning their anger in toward themselves.

WEIGHT CONTROL ADVICE FOR EVERY DOSHA

In addition to the specific recommendations provided above, several principles are common to all doshas.

❋ COOKING WITH WEIGHT LOSS–ENHANCING ❋ KITCHEN SPICES

When you are eating to lose weight, you want to gain flavor so you don't feel deprived and unsatisfied. Herbs and spices in general are a fat-free way to enhance the flavor of all your dishes. To add variety and spice to your cooking, refer to one of the increasing number of Ayurvedic and Indian cookbooks available. Our favorite is *Ayurvedic Cooking for Self-Healing* by Usha Lad and Vasant Lad, available from the Ayurvedic Press in Albuquerque, New Mexico. Using herbs and spices for flavorings in your teas and cooking are not only delicious—they also help you lose weight.

---

1. Eat Appropriate Amounts of Food

The Ayurvedic weight control system is not a diet with strict daily menus. But if you are overweight, you need to eat less food than you are probably used to—certainly less than the typically huge meals you'll find in most American restaurants, which many people have come to think of as "normal" portions.

The easiest way to give yourself reasonable portions is not with measuring spoons and rulers, but with your eyes. According to Ayurveda, each meal should consist of no more than two and a half handfuls of food; if you are trying to lose weight, make that two handfuls; if you are trying to gain, make it three. And, as you learned in "Step 2: Nourish Your Body," your stomach should contain ⅓ solid food and ⅓ liquid, with ⅓ remaining empty so that there is space and energy for digestion.

2. Improve Your Digestive Fire (Agni)

The measures below are specifically designed to rekindle your digestive fire (agni) and burn and eliminate accumulated toxins (ama) so that weight control is easier.

- Before meals: Eat a small piece of finely chopped fresh ginger; or one clove garlic chopped fine, ¼ teaspoon grated gingerroot, and ½

teaspoon lime juice; or 2 teaspoons of fresh radish juice with a pinch of ginger.
· Follow the Ten-Day Ginger Treatment (see page 135) once a month.
· When combining foods, be sure to follow the guidelines on page 37 in Step 2; poor combining will create ama.
· Avoid diet drinks. Sip warm water, ginger tea, or lemon or lime water throughout the day to liquefy ama so it can be more easily eliminated by your body. Take two ounces every half hour.
· Increase the amount of saliva, which contains digestive enzymes, by running your tongue over your teeth several times before a meal.

3. Do a Juice-and-Soup Fast

Many people go on fasts because it's a quick way to jump-start a weight loss program. In Ayurveda, a juice-and-soup fast is recommended because it helps to purify the system and reduce ama. Do this fast one day a week to stabilize kapha and one day every two weeks to stabilize vata or pitta.

Juices · Drink a total of no more than three cups of the following fresh vegetable juices, alone or combined: wheat grass, beets, carrots, kale, parsley. Drink a total of no more than one cup of fruit juice (do not combine).

· · · · · · · · · *V*EGETABLE *S*OUP · · · · · · · ·

(MAKES TWO SERVINGS);

3 cups water
½ cup mung dahl (yellow lentils, available at Indian food stores)
1 medium broccoli spear
3 medium celery stalks, cut up
2 medium zucchini squash, cut up
2 medium carrots, cut up
2 leaves each collard greens, kale, and chard
a few springs parsley
1 tsp. sea salt

Wash mung dahl, bring to a boil in the water, add vegetables and salt. Reduce heat to low and cook, covered, at least ½ hour, or until dahl is soft.

Next, sauté over low heat:

1 T. ghee
1 tsp. whole black mustard seeds
1 tsp. whole cumin seeds
1 tsp. fenugreek seeds

When seeds begin to pop, add:

1 tsp. freshly grated ginger
1½ tsp. freshly ground coriander seeds
½ tsp. turmeric
¼ tsp. ground black pepper

Place the ghee mixture into a blender; add 1 cup cooked soup. Blend for a few seconds, add the rest of the soup, and blend again.

4. Eat the Three Miracle Foods (Milk, Ghee, and Honey)

You don't think of them as diet foods, but according to Ayurveda, these three foods in particular have a potent role to play in weight control.

Milk · Milk is the first natural food, and we get it as infants in the form of mother's milk. Ayurveda believes that our need for the nurturing qualities of milk continues throughout our lives. Milk feeds and nourishes the nervous system, and a healthy nervous system is required for weight control.

Milk is a concentrated source of protein, the building block for tissues, including nerves. In addition, the protein in milk initiates mechanical digestion, so milk is important for treating an exhausted vata. People who gain weight and can't lose it have an exhausted nervous system that is unable to trigger rhythmic body metabolism including the release of digestive enzymes, the churning action of the stomach and the contractions of the intestines. This leads to sluggishness and weight gain.

However, you must never drink plain cold milk, even low-fat or skim milk—this creates ama. It must first be heated or cooked, and it is best consumed along with prescribed spices. The milk then acts as a carrier so the herb or spice is transported into the system to spur a more efficient cycle of cell growth, repair, and energy. Yogurt, another prominently featured food in Ayurveda, is made with cooked milk, and ghee is butter that has been clarified by heating.

The proper way to drink milk is in small amounts, heated, and spiced. Combine ¼ cup milk with the appropriate spice—use your own taste as a guide to the amount, but a pinch is a good place to start. Use saffron for vata, cumin for pitta, and trikatu in low-fat milk for kapha. Nancy soothes her doshas before bedtime with warm almond milk deliciously spiced with vata churna.

Ghee · Many people ask: what is ghee—clarified butter—doing in a weight loss plan? But ghee is actually an essential part of regulating your weight. This light, refined oil lubricates your engine, so digestive enzymes and the food itself are transported easily. Cooking your spices in ghee and then adding that to your vegetable dishes can both be nutritious and delicious. This is not a license to overindulge in butter—if a little is good, more is not necessarily better. Too much ghee, like too much of any oil, will add calories and clog your liver. Add no more than 1 tablespoon a day to the foods you cook. This small amount adds enough lubrication to keep your metabolism moving smoothly and effortlessly along. If I use ghee regularly, I'll lose two or three pounds without changing my diet.

Honey · Honey that has been heated is a powerful tool for weight loss. It dries out the fat and scrapes it off your tissue. That's why I recommend 1 teaspoon a day, in hot water or hot milk. For kaphas I recommend 2 teaspoons of honey with 1 teaspoon of trikatu every day for weight loss. Honey is most effective if you choose the type best suited to your dosha: vata does best with orange blossom honey; pitta with wildflower honey; and kapha with clover honey. Note: Honey should not be cooked; uncooked honey is nectar and cooked honey is a poison. Cooked honey clogs the energy channels. Honey should *not* be combined with equal amounts of ghee.

5. Exercise

It's difficult lose weight and reduce body fat and keep it off unless you are also physically active. Exercise is possibly more important than eating less, according to recent studies. Most people (80 percent) who lose weight through diet alone gain it back within year; most people who also exercise regularly do not gain it back.

Exercise is your greatest ally in weight control for many reasons. It helps you shed pounds because it changes your metabolism, speeding it up so you burn more calories during exercise—and for some time afterward. It prevents your body from slowing down when you reduce your food intake—the body's natural response to what it perceives as impending starvation. Exercise builds muscle mass, and your body needs to burn fat to maintain the muscle; it also trains muscles to burn fat in food for energy so less of it gets stored in your body as fat in the first place. Aerobic exercise in particular is useful because it promotes the loss of fatty tissue rather than lean tissue (muscle) when you lose weight. Exercise also allows you to keep on enjoying food—you don't have to feel deprived. Exercise is in itself pleasurable and improves your mood noticeably, so you are more likely to incorporate it into your lifestyle. Physical activity tones and firms your body, resculpting it so you have a smoother, trimmer contour no matter what your weight. Refer to Step 4 for our discussion of the various types of exercise suitable for each dosha.

6. Pay Attention to the Mind Connection

Although the kapha dosha governs the body's structure and is involved with overweight, it is a troubled vata—the great orchestrator—that is the root cause of most weight problems. The signal that we are hungry emanates from the part of the brain called the hypothalamus; this tiny organ also tells us when we are full. This part of your nervous system might be thought of as your appetite control center. When your nervous system, which is governed by vata, is in a severe state of fight or flight—the stress response—it cannot carry out its other functions.

Certain feelings are able to speed up your metabolism, others slow it down. Remember from "Step 3: Nourishing Your Mind and Spirit" that stress is in the eye of the beholder. Your values, standards, and way of seeing things determine how you react to any given situation. It is important to bring balance in your life by connecting to your body type. You also need to reconnect with your inner self and your present life. Watch yourself, observe yourself, discover yourself—but do not judge yourself because this can set up a pattern of self-loathing and recrimination.

Ask yourself: How do I feel? Am I comfortable physically, mentally, spiritually? When you are comfortable, you usually eat enough, but not too much. When you are uncomfortable—depressed or anxious—you either eat too much or too little. This is one way that your mind influences your weight. Another way is for your thoughts and feelings to remain undigested. You may be in denial and shove the unpleasant feelings away—but they do not go away. They remain inside you, undigested. You get stuck in that emotion, the motion of metabolism stops, and your system becomes clogged with ama.

Ask yourself: Am I hungry for something other than food? If you are not satisfied emotionally or psychologically, you need to look at that—are you using food to fill a void that is best taken care of in other ways? Are you psychologically dependent on food the way some people are dependent on alcohol, caffeine, nicotine, or other drugs? Ayurveda offers several techniques that calm your mind, and help you manage stress and digest emotions. These include breathing exercises, deep relaxation, meditation, yoga, and exercise (see Step 3). I have also found that using therapy that attends to all five senses is a magical approach to weight loss. Therapies that calm vata, the nervous system dosha (see "Five-Senses Therapy" in Step 3), are particularly useful, and others are effective in reducing cravings (see below).

Here's a marvelous way of using your mind to help you start and stay on a weight control program. Read this book, but don't do anything right away. Simply let the knowledge penetrate, give it time to make sense, to click with your innermost being. Use Ayurveda as a framework for seeing yourself as you are—what you are doing now. Watch yourself as if you were watching a film of your life, doing all the things that adversely affect your weight. Then watch another movie in which you see yourself as you could be—getting up at 6 A.M., eating appropriate foods, taking a walk, deep breathing, and so on. Run this second movie in your head every day for two weeks, still without making any changes in your life. Then pick one thing from the new movie and add that to your life with utter resolve and belief behind it. Also take the old movie and run it backward, as if you were erasing it. Do this practice in your mind before and after you meditate, until you have erased the harmful behaviors in your movie and your life and have incorporated several of the new behaviors.

HEALTH AND APPEARANCE PROBLEMS RELATED TO OVERWEIGHT

These health- and appearance-related problems are usually of concern to people who want to lose weight.

Abdominal Bloating

A bloated, distended abdomen—with or without abdominal or intestinal gas—is a terrible feeling and makes you look heftier than you are. This is the cardinal sign of dysfunction of the agni, the digestive fire, and is usually caused by a vata imbalance. In Ayurveda, we describe it as the first sign of an imbalance in the "gastrointestinal consciousness." Bloating occurs when the gastrointestinal tract is unable to split food into the smallest particles and release the nourishing enzymes into the system. To minimize bloating:

- Eat a light diet of primarily vegetables and rice, or Kicharee (page 137). The Ten-Day Ginger Treatment (see page 135) is also recommended.
- Triphala is an Ayurvedic herb that treats the entire digestive tract. Take ½ teaspoon of triphala mixed with ½ cup of warm water every evening at bedtime.
- Emphasize sweet, sour, bitter, and salty foods, spices, and herbs. The summer churna (a combination of herbs and spices, see page 63), plus a little salt and lemon flakes, is an easy way to get all these tastes in the appropriate proportions.
- Use warm sweet, and sour essential oil aromatherapy, such as rose, cloves, cinnamon, basil, and orange.

Cellulite

Cellulite—that infuriating lumpiness that can occur anywhere you have fat deposits, but most commonly around the hips and thighs—is considered to be a kapha disorder. The fat cells' main job is to store energy until it is needed, and then break it down and release it. But when your digestive fire is low for a long time, fat cells accumulate kapha and get clogged. Your fat cells keep expanding like little water balloons until they reach their limits and then divide to form new cells. The bloated extra cells press against the network of collagen under the skin, resulting in the familiar cottage-cheese look. Even if you exercise and lose weight, the cellulite can remain, because the kapha energy is still stuck and the fat in the cells can't break down. It will take several months to see a difference, but there are several things you can do to reduce cellulite:

- Make sure you get enough exercise and do strenuous yoga daily.
- Drink one cup of hot water with one teaspoon fresh grated ginger, three times a day.
- Make a paste of 1 part vacha (calamus), 2 parts guggulu, and ¼ part chitrak; apply to the area with cellulite and let it set for one hour before rinsing off in a warm shower.
- To improve the circulation, massage the area of cellulite for five minutes every day using a silk glove (see Garshana, page 92)
- Massage the cellulite areas with herbal medicated oils. Use narayan oil nightly and neem oil upon arising every day; do not wash off the oil.
- A product called Meda, available through MAPI (see "Mail-Order Suppliers"), reputedly increases the enzymes that break down fat.
- Emphasize bitter, pungent, and astringent foods, spices, and herbs; these tastes are found in the kapha churna (a combination of herbs and spices, see page 63).

Food Cravings, Bingeing, and Overeating

Do you crave rich chocolate . . . or is rich, fatty cheese your nemesis? Perhaps fresh, yeasty bread slathered with butter is your downfall, or that crunchy, salty crispness of potato chips. Whatever the object of your desires, Ayurveda considers cravings to be a mistake of the intellect. Bingeing must surely be misguided, since it usually involves eating large amounts of food, within the space of a couple of hours; you can't stop even though you are full, and you don't even taste the food. Such behavior is spurred by feelings of tension, anxiety, boredom, or loneliness, and the intense burst of eating somehow makes you feel better.

Cravings and binges usually involve fattening foods and junk foods such as ice cream, pudding, cookies, cakes, pastries, crackers, candy, chocolate, peanut butter, nuts, and chips. Eating this way habitually piles on the fat (unless you develop a further eating disorder and also purge through vomiting or frantic exercise). It also produces toxins and clogs your system. Cravings and binges have nothing to do with being physiologically hungry for food. Therefore, just trying to eat sensibly—to eat only when you are hungry and stopping when you are full—is not the answer.

According to Ayurveda, craving and bingeing are due to hunger—but not hunger for food per se. You may be hungry for love or attention or acknowledgment. You don't want the food itself—you want the feeling food gives you. Or you may be starved for the taste—be it sweet, salty, sour, bitter, pungent, or astringent.

As you learned in Step 2, Ayurveda recognizes six different tastes. Taste are considered to be concentrated packets of energy, and each taste is meant to perform a specific function for the brain. Every food, herb, and essential oil has its own vibrational frequency. Tastes have their own frequencies, and these literally ignite certain chemical reactions that activate neurotransmitters and other biochemical processes. When you are getting only three of the six tastes a deficiency is created in your brain chemistry. Unsatisfied, your brain cries out for the other three—in other words, craving can occur because the body does not get a proper amount of all six tastes.

In the United States the most common tastes are sweet, sour, and salty. If you eat the typical diet, your brain misses the other tastes, bitter, pungent, and astringent, as a result. Not only will you be deficient in certain mental functions, but you will also feel emotionally understimulated and dissatisfied. So, the cornerstone in the Ayurvedic approach to controlling cravings and binges is taste therapy. When you give yourself a variety of tastes, you are satisfied and nourished on a physical as well as psychological level. You feel full emotionally and physically so that you don't turn to more food to fill the void.

The late-night snack is a form of overeating unto itself, according to Ayurveda. To understand why, remember that pitta is the dosha responsible for digestion, and the pitta time of day is between the hours of 10 A.M. to 2 P.M. and 10 P.M. to 2 A.M. Therefore, your body is primed to handle food at those times. The daytime pitta period is the best time to eat your largest meal, but the nighttime pitta period is when this dosha is primed to metabolize the food, which is a later stage of digestion. This is a time of high metabolic activity and explains why you may sometimes awaken in the middle of the night feeling hot and sweaty, especially if you have eaten a large dinner. On the other hand, if you are still awake into the high pitta period, you may get the munchies—another mistake of the intellect. So, if you are prone to mindless midnight munching, your best remedy is to go to bed a couple of hours before midnight, to keep your pitta in sync with nature's rhythms.

Taste Therapy · Eat a variety of foods, in all taste categories, according to your dosha and according to the season. Each meal should contain all six tastes, in the correct proportion for your dosha. An easy way to accomplish this is by using the churnas recommended in Step 2 (page 63)—these are collections of spices and herbs designed with the right tastes in the right proportions for the three doshas. Simply get or make the churna appropriate for your dosha and sprinkle some on your food every meal. This is an easy, convenient way to supply your diet with the variety that humans crave. Doing a weekly soup-and-juice fast (see page 164) will also help break the cycle of craving and bingeing. Give this approach three months; that's how long it takes to reregulate your brain chemistry and free yourself from your cravings. And be sure to keep on hand the spiced herbal tea that calms your dosha, and drink a cup whenever you feel a binge or craving coming on.

Aromatherapy · Aromas are tastes for your nose, and sometimes aromatherapy is a more direct and immediate remedy for cravings than taste therapy. For example, if your craving is for vata-calming foods such as soft, sweet, fatty creamy foods or carbohydrates, use aromatherapy essential oils such as basil, orange, rose, geranium, and clove. If you crave crunchy finger foods that require a lot of chewing, such as potato chips, peanuts, popcorn, and crackers, it indicates a pitta-related excitement, frustration, or anger, which responds to essential oils of sandalwood, rose, cinnamon, mint, and jasmine. Kapha-type cravings, which arise out of feelings of depression or lethargy, are usually for stimulants such as coffee or colas or chocolate, which bring you out of your stupor; try instead aromatherapy with stimulating oils such as juniper, eucalyptus, camphor, clove, and marjoram.

Other Tips:

- Take ½ teaspoon triphala with ½ cup warm water at bedtime, daily.
- Combine 5 parts shatavari (Asparagus racemosus), 2 parts tikta, 2 parts kama, and 3 parts guduchi (Tinospora cordifolia); take ¼ teaspoon twice daily, following lunch and dinner.
- For emotional obsessive eating habits, one banana chopped up with one teaspoon of ghee and a pinch of cardamom is very effective.
- Give food your full attention when you are eating so you are satisfied on a psychological level, instead of suddenly noticing your plate is empty and saying, "I can't believe I ate the whole thing!"
- Examine your life to see if stress could be contributing to your excessive eating habits. If so, incorporate one or more of the practices suggested in Step 3, such as breathing exercises, deep relaxation, meditation, or yoga.
- When you feel the urge to eat, try substituting another activity, such as walking or taking a yoga break. You may be eating out of boredom or because you are feeling fidgety. Instead of food what you really crave is a change of scenery or to switch gears.
- Don't prepare large amounts of food. Throw out leftovers, if you are likely to munch on them mindlessly. Leftovers can be a temptation to overeat, and according to Ayurveda, they are unhealthy because they have no life to them and thus create ama.

Water Retention

In Ayurveda, maintaining the proper water balance in the body is kapha's job. Kapha becomes congested when vata becomes imbalanced and stops directing traffic or when pitta is all fired up and the water and earth elements of kapha try to put the fire out. As a result, the lungs, heart, kidney, and other tissues clog up. You feel bloated and heavy, inside and out, as your waterlogged tissues expand and hold water instead of circulating it. Many women complain that they particularly retain water just before and during their menstrual periods, but that bogged-down feeling can strike anytime that kapha becomes sluggish. You need to take measures that stimulate kapha and get the water moving through your system and out of it:

- Pungent, bitter, and astringent tastes should be emphasized; the spring churna (a combination of herbs and spices; see page 63) is an excellent way to introduce these tastes into your everyday diet.
- Essential oils with spicy, warm aromas help stimulate kapha and regulate water in the body.
- Watermelon juice is an effective and delicious natural diuretic; drink one small glass three times a day when this fruit is in season.
- Try herbal therapy. The basic formula is 1 teaspoon triphala with 1 cup warm water before bedtime. In addition, you may take *one* of the following:
  - ★ Make a tea using 1 teaspoon fennel per 1 cup hot water and drink three times a day.
  - ★ Combine ⅓ teaspoon each of punarnava, gokshura, fennel, and ashok with 1 cup hot water; drink three times a day.
  - ★ Take ½ teaspoon of punarnava twice a day, with 1 cup water.

ARE YOU UNDERWEIGHT?

If you would like to gain weight, you are most likely a vata type, or your vata is out of balance. Therefore you need to follow the vata-balancing daily program. Since vata governs the nervous system, make time to incorporate into your life the mind- and spirit-nourishing practices. It is crucial for you to practice stress reduction techniques—if you are underweight, it may be because you burn calories through nervous stress and chaotic emotions. Follow the advice for improving digestion in this chapter—improving digestion will enable your body to better absorb the nutrients it takes in so you gain weight. The following practices should also keep your nervous system on an even keel and stabilize your weight:

General Eating Tips

- Eat regular meals on a regular schedule; eating several small meals during the day is best.
- Always eat cooked foods.
- Eliminate caffeine from your diet.
- Do not watch television when eating. Do not eat while distracted or under stress.
- Eat a variety of foods and avoid excessive eating of one food, especially junk food.
- To improve appetite, chew a piece of lime with a pinch of rock salt before meals.
- Emphasize warm, heavy foods that provide stability, nourishment, and emotional satisfaction.
- Emphasize bitter, pungent, and astringent tastes such as garlic, ginger and fennel, coriander, cumin, dill, mint, peppermint, rose water, saffron, turmeric, ajwain, and those found in the spring churna (a combination of herbs and spices, see page 63).
- Also add the sweet taste to your eating in the form of rice and fresh figs and dates.
- Fruits and vegetables to favor are lemon, lime, pickled mango chutney, kelp, seaweed greens, squashes, yams, and asparagus, and sweet potatoes.
- Pine nuts and almonds are a dense source of nourishment and energy for vatas.
- You may add a little oil to your foods; mustard oil and sesame oil for cooking are the most appropriate for vata.

Other Tips

- For vata-related underweight, drink ½ cup cooked milk with ½ teaspoon jatamansi. Take once a day, between 2 and 6 A.M. or P.M.
- Essential oils with sweet, warm aromas help calm vata and your nervous system, so choose jasmine, clove, rose, cinnamon, and orange scents for your aromatherapy. You may also add three drops of rose aromatherapy oil to two teaspoons of sesame or almond oil; apply this to your wrist and to the back of the head where the skull meets the neck bones (occipital ridge).

STEP 10

Cultivate Your Sexual Charisma

*C*HARISMA IS "A RARE QUALITY OR POWER, A DIVINELY inspired gift or power," according to the dictionary. In Ayurveda it is called *Tej* and is defined as the inner shine radiating from a person that acts as an attractive energy. Sexual charisma—that wondrous primal force—is the most powerful attraction of all.

If cultivating charisma is your goal, outward beauty couldn't hurt—before people can notice your inner radiance, you need to attract their attention. The previous steps in this program will help you do just that, but in a way that is so natural, so expressive of your true inner self that your innate sexual charisma can't help but shine through. Once you've achieved the physical and spiritual grace, vitality, equanimity that are characteristic of charisma, cultivating the sexual part is just the icing on the cake.

In this chapter, you'll learn how to improve your sexual charisma by understanding how your doshas influence your sexual characteristics and what doshas to look for in a mate. We explain how your behavior affects the quality of your sexual relationships, how the five senses can enhance your sexual allure and sexual pleasure, and open the door to an exploration of Tantric sex. Charismatic and dynamic sex appeal is within your grasp; or rather, it is within you already. The goal of Ayurveda is to bring it out and enhance it.

THE ALLURE OF CHARISMA

To be in a state where you are loved and loving, to be sexually exciting and satisfied: this is the ultimate step in achieving inner and outer radiance and beauty—the final reward. Beauty is an empty pleasure unless it enables you to love yourself and others to love you. According to Ayurveda, our fundamental purpose in life is to love. When you realize this and are able to achieve it, your inner love and radiance shines forth and attracts worthy people like honey. Sexual intimacy is but one sublime expression of this love, as well as a means to deepen it.

According to Ayurveda, romantic and erotic love is one of the nine emotions that are natural to life and is a source of rejuvenation, vigor, and beauty. Inner and outer beauty not only attract love, but love then increases this beauty in a never-ending spiral of greater and greater giving and joy. This is why women in love look more beautiful, as do mothers-to-be—they are glowing with the love for and of another. It's no wonder that people write songs and poems about it, search to the ends of the earth to find it, go to great lengths to achieve it, and even risk making fools of themselves once they get it.

Most people say they feel better—wonderful, even—after sex. Perhaps you, too, have noticed that the world seems brighter, your skin glows more radiantly, you have a spring in your step, you sleep better, are more relaxed (or more energized) after a night—or afternoon or morning—of lovemaking.

UNDERSTANDING YOUR SEXUALITY

It's often observed that people who love themselves and who are at ease in their own skins are those who are most likable and lovable. Ayurveda gives you the tools for this, through determining and understanding your doshas, your strengths, and your limitations.

Understanding who you are includes understanding how the different doshas express their true selves through their sexuality. There is a great deal of ancient lore on this subject. The guidelines to follow summarize the ways

---

❋ THE BONDS OF LOVE ❋

Being radiant and attractive can actually be good for your health. Close relationships appear to improve immunity, reduce the risk of heart attack and cancer, and even prevent the common cold. Numerous studies show that a strong and diverse network of social contacts has a physiological effect on your body and your ability to withstand stress. Humans, so far as we know, are unique in this respect to sex: we use it not only for reproduction but also to form emotional bonds, for giving and getting pleasure. Perhaps this is why a satisfying sex life seems to be a way to access your inner energetic source of youth and vitality.

---

in which your doshas influence your sexual characteristics and suggest which doshas tend to make the best matches. See if this information rings true for you so that you can cultivate your sexual strengths and minimize your limitations. Then, consider asking your partner to determine his or her dominant dosha by taking the test in "Step 1: What's Your Body Type?" to see if you're a good match.

- *Vata*: If you are primarily vata, you are a cool, subtle, ethereal, change- able presence. You are quick to feel passion and become attached but are reluctant to commit. You may appear frigid, but you blossom with the right partner. For you, feeling love is more important than the actual act of love. The best doshas for you to partner up with are kapha-pitta, pitta-kapha, and kapha-vata.
- *Pitta*: If you are primarily pitta, you are one hot number—mesmer- izing to others and with strong desires and passions. You burn, but you can also get burned yourself—and you can also burn yourself out. Intense as a lover, you can be jealous, impatient, and lacking in hu- mility around the object of your desire. You need to watch out for becoming overly focused on the sexual act and redirect your emotions away from your sexual organs and toward your heart. This is the way for you to bring love and intimacy to a higher, lasting, more noble and caring, and sublime plane. The best partner for you is one who shares your passion for natural beauty; look to pitta-kaphas, kaphas, and kapha-pittas in a mate.

• *Kapha*: Kaphas are calm, sweet, sensual, earthy, and physically and emotionally voluptuous. If this is your dominant dosha, in love you are shy, cautious, wise, honest, and steady. You take time to fall in love, but when you do, you fall hard. You are deeply committed, romantic and can be possessive. You are a good lover—maternal yet erotic, feminine yet with great stamina. All types are good partners for you, as long as they are strong sexually and otherwise.

BETTER SEX

According to Ayurveda, sex is one of our most divine and powerful natural needs and as long as you are in a state of balance, it should not be repressed. Rather, it should be fully expressed and enjoyed. If you have a partner, you can better use all your senses to enliven and enrich your sexual experiences. If emotional issues are blocking your path—past experiences, cultural conditioning—seek help in removing them.

Dharma

Dharma is another word for "Beauty is as beauty does." Dharma refers to your inner knowledge of what is right and wrong. These are universal codes of behavior, much of which is common sense because they are conducive to your individual well-being as well as the well-being of the society you live in. The primary dharmas are love, faith, purity, compassion, honesty, courage, and devotion. Everyone is born with the knowledge of these dharmas, but you must continue to nurture them if they are to remain alive. When you live your life—including your love life—guided by dharma, all your accomplishments and possessions are infused with happiness and grace.

Making Sex a Total Sensory Experience

All five senses are involved in lovemaking and in the sexual dance that precedes it. Practices included in Five-Senses Therapy can help you open up, liberate, stimulate, and fine-tune your senses so you can derive and give greater pleasure. Preferences for scent, sight, sound, touch, and taste are extremely individualized, so please refer to page 60 in "Step 3: Nourishing

Your Mind and Spirit" for background information. Then use your imagination and creativity to experiment for ways to specifically perk up your sex life using the five senses—yours and your partner's. Here are some ideas to get you started.

- *Appreciate the Scent of Sex.* Fragrance is a potent yet subtle love attractor. Your natural scent may be the most potent of all—pheromones, the natural scent signals we send out, include androstenone, which has a musky smell and drives libido in both men and women. The highest concentrations of pheromones are in the underarm and genital area; androstenone is also found in saliva.
- *Use Aromatherapy.* In addition, you can use aromatic essential oils to enhance your sex appeal and attractiveness or to improve your libido or that of your partner. For your next romantic encounter, light the candles *and* the aromatherapy diffuser. Oils of patchouli, frankincense, musk, and sandalwood are reported to be aphrodisiacs. For frigidity or impotence, use ylang-ylang. Vanilla is also said to increase sexual desire in men.
- *Give a Fragrant Massage.* Another way to take advantage of the power of scent is to add some sandalwood oil to massage oil and give each other a massage; it contains hormones similar to testosterone, the hormone that drives the libido in both men and women.
- *Anoint Yourself.* In India, the use of aromatic oils is a well-established tradition. To get ready for a night of love, a Hindu woman's body is anointed with many different scents to arouse her partner. You can be similarly creative with essential oils; remember to dilute them first with a carrier oil before applying to your skin.
  - ★ jasmine on her hands
  - ★ patchouli on her check and neck
  - ★ amber on her nipples
  - ★ saffron on her feet
  - ★ sandalwood on her inner thighs
  - ★ musk on her pubic area
- *Condition Your Body.* Exercise enhances sexual pleasure in many ways. In a study of sedentary men whose average age was forty-seven, the subjects exercised four times a week. They either took an easy sixty-minute walk or did a more strenuous aerobic workout. At the end of

nine months, both groups said they enjoyed an increase in their sexual desire and pleasure and an enhanced ability to be aroused and achieve orgasm. Those who did the more strenuous activity reported the greatest gains. Exercise improves blood flow throughout the entire body, including the penis, and therefore may improve impotence in men. And the endorphins released by strenuous exercise are believed to make you more receptive to sex.

- *Practice Yoga.* Among the many benefits of yoga are an improved sex life. Think about it: practicing yoga regularly makes all your joints more limber and eases back stiffness and pain so you are able to engage in sex more comfortably and experiment with new positions. Yoga increases your strength and energy, improves your appearance, body shape, tone, and complexion. It is also relaxing and boosts self-confidence and self-esteem while allowing you to feel more at ease, more at home in your body. Many yoga positions are particularly effective for relieving tensions and anxiety, to tone the reproductive organs, balance hormones, and strengthen and tone the pelvic muscles.
- *Get Playful.* There is a smorgasbord of sexual toys available to enhance your sexual pleasure via all the senses—sweet honey dust, tickling feathers, lubricating creams, and so on. These are all in keeping with the philosophy of Ayurveda and are available discreetly through the mail and in small shops in large cities. For example, Living Arts (see "Mail-Order Suppliers" section) sells a Kama Sutra Gift Tin of goodies, a Sensual Aromatherapy Kit, Chocolate Body Paint, and books and videos on sexual massage and Kama Sutra.

Stretching Your Boundaries: Is Tantra for You?

In the Hindu tradition, the esoteric practice of *Tantra* regards sexual energy as a path to spiritual wisdom. For more than two thousand years, India has produced a wealth of erotic literature and art, the most well-known of which is the *Kama Sutra.* Workshops and videotapes, books, and web sites on tantric sexuality are increasing daily, and are an avenue worth exploring if you are looking to vary your technique and move toward a more spiritual form of lovemaking.

The *Kama Sutra* is the earliest surviving example of a Hindu "love manual." A compendium of the social norms and love customs of Northern

---

❦ THE FOOD OF LOVE ❦

Graciousness—goodwill, concern for others, paying attention to the divine nature of the universe, cultivating harmony and comfort—shows in many ways. One of the most fundamental is in preparing and serving food with love and kindness. The sharing of food is traditionally a means to creating an emotion. ("The way to a man's heart is through his stomach.") Avoid projecting your negative emotions onto the food, for they are absorbed and passed on to those who eat it—and if you eat it, back to yourself. Instead, project loving, sensual emotions and see what happens.

India during the time it was written, it places sex within the context of a refined, humane way of life. Although it is most famous for its detailed and graphic descriptions of many love postures, the *Kama Sutra* also includes a discussion of dharma and Ayurvedic aphrodisiacs and potions to increase sexual power.

The *Kama Sutra* also contains some practices that have come to be called Tantra. Tantra, or sacred sex, is becoming an increasingly popular field of study for couples and singles alike. The promise of Tantra is that of more conscious loving, a weaving together of sex and spirituality. According to its proponents, by practicing certain techniques, lovers can intensify passion, prolong sexual encounters, deepen connectedness and intimacy, and reach a higher state of consciousness while locked in sexual embrace. Not only is it presented as a prescription for transcending the boundaries of everyday experience, but as a way of strengthening love, bonds and commitment, and thus of helping relationships survive over the long term.

Ayurveda is based on knowing how your doshas interact with the doshas in nature. So, it is fitting that we end this program with the most intimate interaction of all—the physical and spiritual union with another person. In closing, we'd like to remind you that physical, mental, and spiritual beauty is the most natural and least expensive quality in life, and is by far the most enjoyable experience you can have. We hope your healthy desire to enjoy your natural wealth, opulence, beauty, and sexuality motivates you to create a life that gives you fulfillment and frees you to achieve success in all your endeavors.

APPENDICES

GLOSSARY OF TERMS

abhyanga (ah-bee-YANG-ah): a massage with oil, usually sesame oil.

acid mantle: the thin film covering your skin, consisting of natural oils (sebum), that protects skin from bacteria and helps it retain moisture.

agni (AHG-nee): the digestive fire that helps break down food, feelings, thoughts, and everything you take in through your senses.

ama (AH-mah): impurities remaining after improper digestion; when ama accumulates in the body-mind, these impurities may lead to imbalances in your doshas, symptoms and eventually to disease.

antioxidant: an agent such as vitamin C or E that prevents free radicals from causing damage.

asana (AH-sah-nah): yoga pose.

Ayurveda (ah-your-VAY-dah): the science of life and longevity that is a six-thousand-year-old healing tradition from India.

blackhead: a mixture of oil, dead skin cells, and bacteria that clogs the pore; the black appearance occurs because the material oxidizes.

churna: a combination of powdered herbs and spices.

dharma (DAR-mah): the unwritten code of conduct that makes us aware of the difference between right and wrong.

dosha (DOH-shah): one of the three governing principles or forces that are responsible for controlling the functions of your mind and body. The three doshas are called vata, pitta, and kapha.

exfoliation: removal of dead skin cells from the skin surface; anything used to accomplish this is called an exfoliant.

garshana (gar-SHAH-nah): a dry massage performed with silk gloves.

ghee: clarified butter, used in Ayurveda to lubricate the body-mind and to enhance the effectiveness of herbs and spices.

kapha (KAH-fah): one of the three doshas; it is comprised of water and earth and is responsible for body structure.

malas (MAH-lahs): waste products the body creates.

marma (MAR-mah): one of the 108 points on the skin that are stimulated by Ayurvedic massage and yoga.

nasayana (nah-SAH-yah-nah): inhaling oil to cleanse and lubricate the nasal passages and sinuses.

ojas (OH-jas): the pure end product of proper digestion.

panchakarma (PAHN-cha-KAR-mah): cleansing and purifying techniques used in Ayurveda.

pitta (PIT-tah): one of three doshas; it is comprised of fire and water and is responsible for metabolism.

prakruti (prah-KROO-tee): your essential nature, as expressed by the proportion of the three doshas that you were born with.

prana (PRAH-nah): the life-force, or breath; similar to chi in Chinese medicine.

Pranayama (PRAH-nah-YAH-mah): breathing exercises.

rasayana (RAH-sah-YAH-nah): remedies and tonics based on combinations of herbs and spices.

sadhanas (sad-HAH-naz): a set of daily practices that are unique to each dosha that keep you in tune with nature and thus keep your prakruti balanced.

tri-dosha (TRY-doh-shah): the three doshas together; often refers to a remedy or practice that stabilizes all three doshas simultaneously.

vata (VAH-tah): one of the three doshas; it is comprised of air and space and is responsible for movement.

vikruti (veh-KROO-tee): your current condition; the ratio of your three doshas that fluctuates along with your health.

yoga: a practice of movement (asanas) and breathing (pranayama) that dissolves the separation between mind and body; it prepares the practitioner for meditation as well as encourages the nervous system, endocrine system, internal organs, and muscles to function at their optimum level.

Glossary of Ayurvedic Herbs and Spices

In Ayurveda, certain herbs, spices, and essential oils derived from them are applied directly to the skin to clean it and keep it healthy and attractive. Also, certain herbs and spices are used medicinally for a short period of time to treat specific conditions. The following herbs are recommended in Steps 4 and 5, to treat specific skin and hair conditions, and in Step 9 to affect your appetite and metabolism and thus stabilize your weight. (See "Mail Order Suppliers," page 190)

Ashwagandha (Winter cherry) is used for its ability to rejuvenate, tone, and promote vitality and sexual energy.

Brahmi is the Indian name for the herb also known as gotu kola. It is used for its ability to rejuvenate and to help heal wounds and relieve skin inflammation.

Guggula compounds come in several types, each made with the resin of guggul, a relative of myhrr. They are used primarily to treat nervous system disorders, and to dissolve fat in the body.

Neem comes from the leaves of the neem tree. A multipurpose herb, it is used for healing chronic and acute skin problems and is particularly effective for pitta problems.

Trikatu is another combination mainstay and consists of black pepper, long pepper, and dry ginger; its uses include indigestion, cough, low agni, and weak digestive fire.

Triphala is a traditional herbal cleansing compound that is used as an all-around tonic. It helps balance all three doshas and is composed of three fruits in dried, powdered form, hence the name, tri-phala. The three fruits are *amalaki* (pitta-cooling and balancing), *haritaki* (vata-warming and balancing), and *bibhitaki* (kapha-stimulating and balancing). Triphala is the mainstay in treating and preventing many conditions; unlike other Ayurvedic herbal formulas, triphala may be taken for several months. Triphala is generally taken mixed with warm water and consumed as a tea upon arising or before bedtime.

Turmeric is the most potent and versatile medicinal herb used in Ayurveda. Known as *haldi* (HAL-dee) in Sanskrit, it is considered sacred and is said to act as an all-around tonic that prevent disease and "cures the whole person."

When taken orally, it reduces gas and helps strengthen digestion by maintaining the "good" bacteria of the intestine and tonifying this organ. It is also reputed to help reduce stress and anxiety. Turmeric is a pungent, bitter astringent, warming and is beneficial for all doshas. However, it does aggravate pitta, so it is important to choose the right dosage for yourself. I would recommend that vata types start with ¼ teaspoon, pittas start with ⅛ teaspoon, and kapha with ½ teaspoon in water, tea, or food.

Shatavari (Asparagus racemosus) is a female toner for the reproductive organs and is often combined with licorice and turmeric.

Precautions for Taking Herbs: If you are presently taking medications, or are under medical treatment for a specific medical condition, it is essential to consult your health professional before administering Ayurvedic medicines. Some herbs should be avoided or used under the guidance of a professional if you have a chronic illness or diagnosed medical problem. Use caution when using herbs. In some people certain herbs may cause undesirable reactions. Begin with the lowest recommended dosage and increase gradually as needed.

Glossary of Skin Care Ingredients

The following ingredients are used in "Step 4: A Beautiful Face Every Day" and "Step 5: Beauty Secrets for Your Skin and Hair."

Base oils: to make the moisturizers and massage oils, you mix essential oils with gentle base oils or carrier oils. We recommend that you use pure "cold-pressed" or "expeller-pressed" organic oils, available in health food stores and many supermarkets. Oils from conventionally grown seeds may contain residues of pesticides and fertilizers that enter your body through the skin.

Essential oils: Essential oils combined with the recommended base oils are powerful agents, and a little goes a long way in helping to hydrate the skin, balance the doshas, lubricate and nourish the skin, and rejuvenate cells. Some people are allergic or hypersensitive and thus, we are intentionally conservative in the proportion of essential oils to base oils. If you prefer a stronger scent, you may gradually add a little more essential oil until your nose is satisfied.

Honey: Many remedies for dry skin and wrinkles include honey, which is a known humectant—that is, it attracts and holds moisture, which in turn plumps up the skin and smoothes out wrinkles. In Ayurveda, honey is known as a *yogahavi,* which means that it has the ability to enhance anything it is combined with; thus it increases the penetration of the following remedies and encourages tissue assimilation. Honey is most effective if you choose the type best suited to your dosha: vata does best with orange blossom honey; pitta with wildflower honey; and kapha with clover honey.

Turmeric powder: Discussed above as a medicinal herb, turmeric is also traditionally used for general skin care. We recommend that for beautiful skin you take turmeric daily, either in food or in capsule. Turmeric is a natural antibiotic and antiviral herb, so it is very cleansing and it is therefore applied externally to treat skin problems and to heal wounds. Note when using turmeric externally that you need to be aware that turmeric can stain if allowed to stay on too long. Thoroughly wash your hands and rinse the sink after using powdered turmeric.

Water: Today's tap water contains chemicals that kill harmful microorganisms, dissolve soap, and protect your teeth but may not be best for your skin. If possible, after cleansing, give your skin a final rinse with bottled or filtered water, and use this also to moisten your skin before applying a moisturizer. Temperature counts, too—according to Ayurveda, you should never use hot water on your face—cool or lukewarm is best.

MAIL-ORDER SUPPLIERS

You may order the Ayurvedic products mentioned in this book through the mail from the following suppliers. Most will send a free catalog upon request.

Kaya Ayurveda Institute
2200 County Center Drive Suite B
Santa Rosa, CA 95423
707-527-7313
Dr. Helen Thomas's Ayurvedic product line is available through the mail; the line, called Kayaveda, consists of aromatherapy, herbs, churnas (herb and spice combinations), light gels, oils, medicated ghees.
email: drst@concentric.net
Website: Kayaveda.com

Bazaar of India
1810 University Avenue
Berkeley, CA 94703
800-261-SOMA
Wholesale and retail herbs, herbal formulas, teas, oils.

Herbalvedic Products—Ayur Herbal Corporation
P.O. Box 6054
Santa Fe, NM 87502
505-889-8569

Infinite Possibilities
60 Union Avenue
Sudbury, MA 01776
800-858-1808
Educational books, audio and videotapes; vedic music CDs and tapes; balancing teas, seasonings, herbal formulas, aromatherapy oils, and massage oils; tongue scrapers.

Living Arts
P.O. Box 2939
Venice, CA 90291-2939
800-254-8464
Clothing, accessories, and instructional media to help you explore yoga, meditation, and massage.

Living Arts
All manner of high-quality items designed to help you relax, meditate, develop spiritually. Books, tapes, CDs, yoga, Tai Chi accessories and clothing.
1-800-525-9515

Lotus Brands
P.O. Box 325
Twin Lakes, WI 53181
414-889-8561

Lotus Herbs
1505 42nd Avenue, Suite 19
Capitola, CA 95010
408-479-1667

MAPI (Maharishi Ayur-veda Products International)
1334 Pacific Avenue
Forest Grove, OR 97116
800-634-9057
Sole distributor of Maharishi Ayur-veda products, an extensive line of herbs, teas, oils, food supplements, incense, and more.

Melanie Sachs
"Invoking Beauty with Ayurveda" Seminars
214 Girard Blvd. N.E.
Albuquerque, NM 87106
505-265-4826
Offers training in Ayurvedic facial massage and beauty practices.

AYURVEDIC AND RELATED ORGANIZATIONS

Contact the following if you wish to receive professional panchakarma treatments, information on Ayurvedic courses, and referrals to Ayurvedic practitioners:

American Institute of Vedic Studies
David Frawley, Director
P.O. Box 8357
Santa Fe, NM 87504
505-983-9385

The Ayurveda Center of Santa Fe
1807 Second St. Suite 20
Santa Fe, NM 87505
505-983-8898

The Ayurvedic Institute and Wellness Center
P.O. Box 23445
Albuquerque, NM 87192-1445
505-291-9698
Conducts an Ayurveda correspondence course by noted Ayurveda expert
Dr. Robert Svoboda; also publishes a newsletter.

The Chopra Center for Well Being
7590 Fay Avenue, Suite 403
La Jolla, CA 92037
619-551-7788
Conducts various educational programs related to Ayurveda including
workshops and training in meditation, as well as Ayurvedic diagnosis and
treatment programs.

College of Maharishi Ayur-Ved
Maharishi International University
1000 N. Fourth Street, DB1155
Fairfield, IA 52557-1155
Offers training program in Maharishi Ayur-Ved.

Lotus Ayurvedic Center
4145 Clares Street Suite D
Capitola, CA 95010

Victoria Stern, N.D.
P.O. Box 1814
Laguna Beach, CA 92652
714-494-8858

Tree of Life Health Practice
Gabriel Cousens, MD
P.O. Box 778
Patagonia, AZ 85624
520-394-5219
The holistic health center offers a week-long panchakarma cleansing and rejuvenation program.

AYURVEDIC COSMETIC COMPANIES

Bundi Facial Skin Care
A Division of Pratima, Inc.
109–17 72nd Road, Lower Level
Forest Hills, NY 11375
718-268-7348

Shivani Products
Devi Inc.
P.O. Box 377
Lancaster, MA 01523
800-237-8221

Dr. Singha's Mustard Bath and More
Natural Therapeutic Center
2500 Side Cove
Austin, TX 78704
800-856-2862

Source School of Tantra
P.O. Box 69
Paia, Maui, Hawaii 96779
808-572-8364
fax (808) 572-8622
e-mail: tantra@mauigateway.com
Addresses for Caroline and Charles Muir, who run workshops on tantric sex.

Swami Sada Shiva Tirtha
Ayurvedic Holistic Center
82A Bayville Ave.
Bayville, NY 11709
516-628-8200

Tantra.com
P.O. Box 1818
Sebastopol, CA 95472
e-mail: e-sensuals@tantra.com;
for catalog only: catalog@tantra.com
1-800-9-tantra (1-800-982-6872) or U.S.A. (707) 823-3063
Fax: (707) 829-9542
A worldwide forum presenting information, discussion, and unique products relating to Tantra, sexual enhancement, and Sacred Sexuality.

TEJ Beauty Enterprises, Inc.
(an Ayurvedic beauty salon owned by Pratima Raichur, founder of Bindi)
162 W. 56th St. Room 201
New York, NY 10019
212-581-8136

Natural Health Magazine
Publishes articles on Ayurveda and other natural approaches; publishes listings and advertisements for suppliers of Ayurvedic products.

Yoga Journal
Publishes articles and advertisements for yoga and Ayurveda-related products and services such as audio and videotapes, courses, sticky mats, and props such as bolsters, belts, and blocks.

FURThER READING

There are many excellent books on Ayurveda for those who wish to delve more deeply into this health system. The following are highly recommended.

Bruning, Nancy, and Thomas, Helen. *Ayurveda: The A–Z Guide to Healing Techniques from Ancient India*. New York: Dell, 1997.

Chopra, Deepak. *Ageless Body, Timeless Mind: The Quantum Alternative to Growing Old*. New York: Harmony Books, 1993.

———. *Creating Health: How to Wake Up the Body's Intelligence*. Boston: Houghton-Mifflin, 1991.

———. *Perfect Health*. New York: Harmony Books, 1990.

———. *Perfect Weight*. New York: Three Rivers Press, 1994.

———. *Quantum Healing:Exploring the Frontiers of Mind-Body Medicine*. New York: Bantam, 1989.

Frawley, David. *Ayurvedic Healing: A Comprehensive Guide*. Salt Lake City, Utah: Passage Press, Morris Publishing, 1989.

Iyengar, B.K.S. *Light On Pranayama*. New York: Crossroad Publishing Company, 1987.

Lad, Vasant. *Ayurveda: The Science of Self-Healing*. Santa Fe, NM: Schocken Press, 1984.

Lad, Usha, and Vasant Lad. *Ayurvedic Cooking for Self-Healing*. Albuquerque NM: Ayurvedic Press, 1994.

Moore, Thomas. *The Soul of Sex*. New York: HarperPerennial, 1998.

Muir, Charles, and Caroline Muir. *Tantra: The Art of Conscious Loving*. San Francisco: Mercury House, 1987.

Sachs, Melanie. *Ayurvedic Beauty Care: Ageless Techniques to Invoke Natural Beauty*. Twin Lakes, WI: Lotus Press, 1994.

Scheibner, Adrianna, M.D. *The Essence of Beauty: An Indispensable Guide to Living in Health and Beauty for People Who Care About the Quality of Life*. Los Angeles: A & A Pubisher & Distributors, 1994.

Svoboda, Robert E. *Prakruti: Your Ayurvedic Constitution*. Albuquerque, NM: Goecom Limited, 1988.

Tiwari, Maya. *Ayurveda: A Life of Balance*. Rochester, VT: Healing Arts Press (1995).

INDEX

ABOUT THE AUTHORS

Dr. Helen Thomas is a doctor of chiropractic who has studied Ayurveda since 1987 with Deepak Chopra, Vasant Lad, Raju, and other leading Ayurvedic physicians. Dr. Helen Thomas has established the Kaya Ayurveda Center in Santa Rosa, California. The Center provides comprehensive and holistic techniques that synthesize chiropractic, Ayurveda, NAET, Bodywork, and Bioenergetics. She is the co-author, with Nancy Pauline Bruning, of *Ayurveda: The A–Z Guide to Healing Techniques from Ancient India*. Dr. Thomas is a popular lecturer and teacher and gives frequent workshops and seminars on Ayurveda to health professionals and the general public.

Nancy Pauline Bruning is a writer specializing in health, fitness, and the environment. She is the author or co-author of more than twenty books, including *Ayurveda: The A–Z Guide to Healing Techniques from Ancient India* (Dell, 1997), *The Real Vitamin and Mineral Book* (Avery, 1997), *The Mend Clinic Guide to Natural Medicine for Menopause and Beyond* (Dell, 1997), *Healing Homeopathic Remedies* (Dell, 1996), *The Natural Health Guide to Antioxidants* (Bantam, 1994), *Breast Implants: Everything You Need to Know* (Hunter House, 2nd edition, 1995), and *Coping with Chemotherapy* (Ballantine, 2nd edition, 1993). She also writes articles for national magazines and patient-education brochures. Nancy Pauline Bruning is a native New Yorker who currently lives in San Francisco.